in good hands

a guide to seeking and receiving massage

Debra Ty

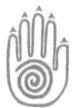

With a Foreword by Carole Osborne

In Good Hands: A Guide to Seeking and Receiving Massage
Printed by CreateSpace.com
Printed in the United States of America

Cover photograph of leaf and author's photo © 2011 by Ron Pierce

Edited and copyedited by Ignatius Aloysius

Cover design/Imaging by Ignatius Aloysius and
Cynthia Kerby (http://www.trueideas.net)

Category: Self-help/Health & Wellness

Some of the names and details used in this book have been changed to
protect the privacy of the people who shared their stories with the author.

ISBN: 1466414669
ISBN-13: 9781466414662
Library of Congress Control Number: 2011918558
CreateSpace, North Charleston, SC

This book is printed on acid-free paper

Dedication

In memory of my dad, Herb Krivacs; my aunt, Marge Stender; my good friend, Bette Goodrich; and my furry feline companion, teacher, and healer, Felicidad.

Contents

PART ONE

SEEKING MASSAGE: How to find the best match in a therapist, type of massage, and environment

Chapter 1: Finding the Right Therapist for You

Chapter 2: Massage Environments

Chapter 3: Interviewing the Massage Therapist

Chapter 4: Most Common Types of Massage/Bodywork (Techniques, Benefits, and Cautions)

Chapter 5: You Want Massage but Cannot Afford It (Ways to Afford Massage)

PART TWO

RECEIVING MASSAGE: Now that you know who you want and what you want, what do you do when you get there?

Contents

Chapter 11: Post-Massage Care (Invest in Your Investment)

Chapter 12: Wrapping It Up (Scheduling Your Next Massage, Tipping, and Cancellations)

Chapter 13: Integrating Massage with Alternative and Conventional Medicine

Chapter 14: More Massage Stories

Adrian's story   Christi's story

Mark's story   Sheri's story

Aletha's story   Teresa's story

Rachielle's story   Tom's story

Susan's story   Marilyn's story

Tara's story   Kathy's story

Serge's story   Patrice's story

Ray's story   Cecelia's story

Mark B's story (The Good Soldier)

Contents

Acknowledgments

To Rick Tyhurst, the first person to affirm my love of massage, who then encouraged and supported me in training fully and in launching my career.

To Lorna B. and other health practitioners at the Sparks Holistic Health Center in Nevada: You gave me a good start on my path to alternative health. And to all practitioners since then who have treated me and nurtured me.

To the International Professional School of Bodywork (IPSB), and The University for Humanistic Studies (UHS), for excellent holistic education which included Tai Chi. Special thanks to Nancy Ursuliak, you taught what you embodied, disclosing your humanness in the process.

To Marla McBride for hours and years of fulfilling bodywork exchanges, imprinting what is most valuable, and for supporting me and stretching me in so many ways.

To Jill Badonsky for getting me started with this book; and to Ignatius Aloysius for deepening and expanding it, and for seeing it through to completion.

To everyone who shared a story within these pages: Thank you for your honest disclosures.

To Goddess power: Dorothy Badeau, Cathy DiSalvo, Caron Grandon, and Michele Muska.

To my moon-lodge sisters: Patrice Archuleta, Ann Hardy, Nancy, Diane, Jan Lawson, Elva Younkin, Mary O., and Eleanor Hovaten. And, of course, to James for his behind-the-scenes support.

To Northeast of Normal, Sethians—you know why.

To my Mastermind partners, Catherine Halmay and Lori Bloom. For our likenesses and differences, laughter and tears, weekly three year commitment to ourselves and to each other, and discussing everything, including the writing of this book.

To Jeanne Walsh at Brooks Memorial Library in Brattleboro Vermont for help with research.

To Sandra Marak, a true professional in our field, who continually improves the discipline through compassionate words and touch, and who offered her editing, feedback, and *A Sacred Mission* poem; as well, thank you to so many of you over the years who have contributed your unique perspective on massage.

To Carole Osborne, for pioneering our field with a bright torch, for being one of my first mentors in massage, and for bestowing my book with your foreword.

Every single person beneath my massaging hands has inspired this book and the evolution of my expertise. Who knows fully what the synergy of client and practitioner co-creates? My heartfelt gratitude to all of you, and to the creator of us all.

Lastly, I wish to acknowledge my family, friends, and associates—you have a special place in my life and in this book.

Foreword

By the time we are adults, most of us generally know what to expect when we visit our doctors or need medical tests or treatments. Decades of medical television dramas plus our and our families' health crises have made many surgeries familiar procedures. When we reluctantly settle into the dentist's chair, it's not because we don't know how the filling of a tooth will proceed. X-rays, mammograms, and our physical check-ups are routine for most of us for whom modern allopathic medical care is so readily accessible.

But therapeutic massage and bodywork is different; many folks just aren't quite sure what they are about to experience or what is expected of them when they reach a massage table or chair. Somatic practices of massage and bodywork have only recently begun to blossom into recognizable forms of healthcare. Despite high professional standards, our skilled and caring therapists have suffered "mistaken identity" as prostitutes or quacks, scaring off multitudes and attracting others who leave disappointed. Until the last twenty years or so, a therapeutic massage has been mostly unavailable to a broad spectrum of populations. When contemplating the intimacy of therapeutic massage and bodywork sessions, many people need reassurances and information to feel comfortable and increase the benefit of the work.

With decades of experience conveying the essence of bodywork to her own clients, Debra Ty is proficient, thorough, and sensitive in her providing helpful information, from how to find the right therapist, common practice protocols, and types of therapeutic methods to how to maximize session outcomes and how to wrap up a session with a massage therapist. She covers all aspects of being a massage therapy client.

This book is a natural reflection of who Debra is as an individual and as a therapist. From the first time I worked with her as a student attending the International Professional School of Bodywork in San Diego, she has impressed me with her grounded presence, direct and warm demeanor, and bright intelligence. Always committed to the highest standards of practice and procedures, she has enjoyed a thriving practice in many locations. Why? Of course she is a gifted therapist with sensitive hands, compassionate heart, and focused mind. In addition, she has an easy ability to meet people where they are and gently yet decisively guide them to a clearer place, just as she does in this book.

For those of you considering massage therapy or bodywork, this book will answer your questions and help to ensure that you are in good hands. Debra's thoughtful yet simple advice will maximize the potential benefit from your sessions. Let her reassure and guide you to the world of therapeutic massage and bodywork.

≈

For therapists committed to informed and participatory practice, using this book will improve your effectiveness and client communications. Whether you melt through fascia, mobilize joints, stimulate energy meridians, or gracefully glide the body's slopes, you will find your clients are more prepared and participatory in their sessions after reading this book. Distribute a copy to prospective clients and referral sources, and watch your appointment book fill. Expect to enjoy improved session outcomes when you lift your practice to a new level of satisfaction for you and your clients.

≈

Carole Osborne is author of *Pre- and Perinatal Massage Therapy* and *Deep Tissue Sculpting*. She was also named the 2008 American Massage Therapy Association National Teacher of the Year.

My Story

Many people ask me why I chose massage as a profession, and I answer "My own back problems led me to massage." In truth, by the age of twenty-six I was gradually losing the ability to do the activities I enjoyed, like hiking, biking, backpacking, and dancing.

I sought help at Excalibur Holistic Center in Sparks, Nevada, and after my first visit which began with a general practitioner, I knew I had encountered a different approach to health—one that involved my physical body, emotions, state of mind, and lifestyle. At Excalibur, I was welcomed and heard on many levels, something I had not experienced before that first visit; and although this exposure was rare for me, I was about to experience it again with each specialist that my general practitioner recommended: a naturopath, chiropractor, psychotherapist, Feldenkrais practitioner, and massage therapist. These professionals related to me and addressed all levels of my being, just as my general practitioner had also done.

The chiropractor, however, was unable to move my skeleton because my muscles were too tight. The naturopath prescribed supplements and homeopathic remedies, after talking to me extensively about what stressed my life and how I responded to the stress; but the supplements, remedies, and my personal process worked minimally—or what I would later learn is that all this only stirred my emotions and caused them to ripen. When I landed in the psychotherapist's office, I thought the specialist and I made a timely match; and although he helped me tremendously, the tension in my muscles persisted.

About this time, a massage therapist named Lorna joined the staff at Excalibur, and my life was about to change in many ways. Lorna helped my muscles to relax through massage, and she taught me to listen to my body, mind, and emotions; her work reinforced my psychotherapy sessions. Above all, she poignantly modeled a profession I would later join, for I knew that I simply had to give others back their lives as she was giving my life back to me.

≈

My first massage with Lorna was perfect imprinting, and it began with a hot tub in the same room in which I was to receive my massage. Submerged in hot water, I gazed through a steamy window into a colorful garden, and my descent into relaxation made me feel as though I were part of an Impressionist painting. The scent of fresh mint leaves permeated the air, and hanging green plants encircled the room. I thrived in the warmth and moisture. Tiny colored bottles filled a smaller window, and flannel sheets on the massage table beckoned me, as the timer to the hot tub switched off and I slowly rocked back to stillness. Lorna appeared, offering a glass of cold water with a lemon slice. I was more relaxed than I had been in a long time, and the massage had not yet begun. In fact, being cared for in this way was as much a relief to me as it was a challenge, because I did not receive the massage as easily as I had expected. Although I tried to relax, my muscles did not always respond, but when they did, my massage was blissful. There were other times when I thought I was relaxed, until Lorna made me aware of my tension and instructed me to breathe and let my tension go.

I felt very different at the end of my first session—light, giddy, and taller. I floated out of Lorna's office, only to drag myself back to her many times afterwards. The effects of my massage would vary from my being rested, tired, energized, emotional, and grounded. Eventually, I began arriving for my massage with less stress and tension, and this helped me to respond to the pressure under Lorna's hands. Instead of resisting, I yielded, and my visits became more pleasurable than painful. Combined with psychotherapy, supplements, and chiropractic care, massage primarily resolved my back problems; it freed me from my muscle-bound straitjacket, which immobilized my body, mind, emotions, and spirit.

≈

One weekend, Lorna taught a massage class and I attended it with a friend. I reveled in a new world of touch and sensation, of feeling muscles change beneath my hands. I even enjoyed the test Lorna gave: I was to venture into her basement library, find one new stroke that she did not teach us, and use it for our hands-on exam. While looking for new strokes, I became so interested in what I was reading that I forgot I had a test to complete. Lorna's workshop stimulated my thirst for more knowledge, and her lifestyle as a massage therapist and teacher inspired me to do the same.

I thrived in this environment of patience and yielding, and of learning and healing, where touch and intimacy were expressed and received appropriately. I found that giving massage was just as desirable as receiving it, and learned that massage provides a connection to the self and to one's environment while helping us feel a kinship with one another; moreover, I did not experience these same qualities in my corporate work setting. The world, I believe, needs more healing and connectedness, and I was inspired to give it.

For twenty-four years, I have been giving back through massage, and I continue to do so even today. Being a massage therapist is a rich endeavor; by helping others obtain a better quality of health and lifestyle, I am inspired to do the same for myself. Actually, I find it difficult to tune into a client energetically and intuitively if my blood sugar is imbalanced by my eating excess chocolate—my vice—or by my eating improperly in general. I must also be fit and cannot depend on my massage workday alone to keep me in good form; I must be stronger than my day's work, and for this I rely on Tai Chi mostly. The very act of massaging is both a physical workout as well as a meditation, which helps me to stay present in each moment and in quiet concentration.

I first learned Tai Chi at massage school: the International Professional School of Bodywork (IPSB) in San Diego, California. Tai Chi is a required course here, because it teaches proper body mechanics for working around the massage table, and because it builds endurance and flexibility. Tai Chi also teaches you how to receive energy while giving energy, so that you do not deplete yourself in the process.

In addition to Tai Chi for a fit, relaxed, and healthy lifestyle, I practice *mindfulness meditation* and apply it as a way of life. I also continue to do what I learned was good for me at Excalibur Holistic

Center: I receive massage, chiropractic, acupuncture, and other alternative methods that fine-tune my entire system—body, mind, emotion, and spirit. Receiving this care makes me a better massage therapist and person, and it helps to keep me in touch with my clients' perspectives, thereby maintaining the balance of giving and receiving.

Introduction

My career in massage (or bodywork) began in 1987, and during that time I have worked in several environments, which include a private practice (in my home offices and in professional settings), outcalls (massage provided in settings outside my office, such as a client's home or office), massage in a chiropractor's office, a day spa, hair salon, and medical center. I have also provided chair massage at corporations, airports, conventions, art shows, and more; but no matter where I gave people their first massage, many would sigh with deep regret and say, "Why didn't I do this years ago?" My heart went out to them and to others who had not yet received their first massage and were missing out. So I began asking: What reasons did people have that kept them from receiving massage sooner? And I heard many prevailing worries and concerns such as the following: "I didn't know what to expect or what to do," or "I do not know the different types of massage or what to ask for," and "The intimate environment made me uncomfortable," even "I did not want anyone to see me naked," and "I am overweight, embarrassed about my body." The honest disclosures continued, and I heard other statements like "It would be odd having a strange man or woman touch me," and "I was afraid I would get an erection," or "I am very ticklish," and "It seemed like such a decadent, selfish thing to spend money on." As well, others said, "I thought my spouse would be jealous," and "I have heard it is painful." All responses touched on common themes related to massage and the unanswered confusions surrounding this healing practice.

My desire to address these concerns became the conception of this book, and writing it was my compassionate act to guide people sooner than later to the world of massage. For those of you already receiving massage, I hope you discover more ways to enjoy your sessions.

It is my belief that massage is a vehicle for peace, because it instills tranquility in the receiver and because notions of conflict and retaliation do not dwell in the post-massaged person. So let peace begin within.

Part One

SEEKING MASSAGE: How to find the best match in a therapist, type of massage, and environment

Chapter 1:
Finding the Right Therapist for You

Referrals: Begin where you place your trust

When seeking a referral, follow the yellow brick road and begin where people you know have placed their trust. Ask your day-to-day contacts—family members, neighbors, friends, and co-workers—or consult your hairstylist, esthetician, and manicurist, and even ask the waitstaff at your favorite restaurants and people at your gym or spa. You may also obtain a referral through your current healthcare professionals such as doctors, chiropractors, acupuncturists, nutritionists, and dentists.

Referrals from these sources offer a name and number of someone who is trustworthy, and often include information regarding environment, location, type of massage, and possibly the perceptions and experiences of the person making the recommendation.

The Yellow Pages

Let your fingers do the walking, indeed. Individuals, groups, organizations, and schools offering massage list themselves under "Therapeutic Massage" or "Massage" in the Yellow Pages, and make available different types of massage through this source. Practitioners do their best to attract clients that suit their services.

The World Wide Web

A wealth of information exists on the Internet, and the subject of massage is no exception. Most organizations' Web sites have a link to help you find a therapist in your area. If you do not know of a specific organization or individual to search for, you may do a general search.

Find a Massage Therapist

An easy way to get started is to type, "Find a Massage Therapist" in the search engine for whichever browser you use, such as Google, Yahoo, and Bing. This will provide you with a listing of massage organizations and individuals. When you select a listing, it will lead you through the process of finding a therapist. You will be asked questions such as the name of a therapist and the location where you would like to receive your massage. If you do not have a therapist in mind, type a keyword for the type of massage you would like to receive; if you do not know what type of massage to ask for, you may want to refer to the section in Chapter 4 called Most Common Types of Massage/Bodywork (Techniques, Benefits, and Cautions).

Or, you may simply state your need for their services, such as, back pain, muscle spasms, relaxation, and so on. The therapist will know how to help you from here.

When filling in the location field as to where you would like to receive a massage, I suggest you find a therapist closest to the destination where you will return to after your massage, as you will no doubt be relaxed and want to remain so. For instance, you may have scheduled your massage after work and intend to go home afterwards; in this case, provide your home address and plan on fulfilling any stressful commute before receiving your massage.

≈

The "find a massage therapist" service also includes a toll free number. By calling this number, someone will provide a list of massage therapists in your area. Additionally, to help you find the best match for your needs, the operator can look up the type of massage you desire and provide the therapists' years of experience for that category.

Wellness Clinics, Open Houses, Massage Schools, and Health Food Stores

Several massage schools, wellness clinics, and health food stores offer lectures and demonstrations of massage routinely or during special events. This is an opportunity for you to meet professionals in their field and hear them discuss their massage techniques and processes; it is also a chance to sample their work. Many speakers ask for a volunteer to demonstrate their work, and some venues have a separate room or area where additional massage therapists offer a sampling of their work for little or no charge. This is a good way for you to meet potential therapists and experience their work, as you may decide to have future sessions with one of them.

Health food stores generally have community bulletin boards where you will find a list of local alternative health practitioners, services, and workshops. In addition, employees at these stores may have experienced the work of listed practitioners and can provide more information.

Medical Extension Plans

Many medical insurance plans now offer a medical extension plan, which is merely a listing of practitioners who have discounted their fees for this purpose. This extension plan is not the same as the services covered by your insurance provider, and the two plans are distinct from one another. The extension plan was developed by insurance companies that do not cover alternative health services such as massage, and the plan works like this: The insurance provider contacts interested massage therapists who agree to discount their fees 10%–25% for insurance plan members. Your insurance provider then suggests a list of participating massage therapists you can call. *However, the only involvement your insurance company has with this transaction is providing you with the names of therapists.* You pay the therapist the discounted fee once you receive your massage. When scheduling your massage, it would be wise to confirm the massage therapist's participation in the extension plan and the affiliated fee that you hope to pay.

Considering the Gender of Your Massage Therapist

Massage therapy is a female-dominated profession, according to AMTA's 2009 industry survey, which shows that women make up eighty-five percent of the workforce, a percentage that has remained consistent for a number of years. Nevertheless, you may choose to state your preference for a male or female massage therapist; however, when scheduling your massage through a spa or center that employs more than one therapist, you will be entrusted with a practitioner according to his or her availability, while the facility does its best to honor any specific requests from you.

Keep in mind the essential attributes of male massage therapists; they may impart more pressure through their hands with greater ease for those desiring this experience, and this added pressure is well suited for sports massage, deep tissue, and other types of massage requiring more physical strength. In no way do I imply that female massage therapists are not suited for massage requiring strength; I merely provide information that expands your options to receive massage as a client from both male and female therapists. Female clients of mine who prefer male therapists, disclosed their reasons for requesting a male therapist and agreed that women with minimal interaction with men find massage with a male therapist as an appropriate way to be with the male perspective. Furthermore, my female clients appreciated the development of intuitiveness and sensitivity in their male therapists.

Points worth rubbing in:
1. Seek and ask. There are many resources available to you.
2. The right massage therapist and location is out there for you right now.

Chapter 2:
Massage Environments

There are several environments to receive massage, and your referral source can inform you of what to expect, or you can ask relevant questions when you call to schedule an appointment with a therapist. The following possibilities will help you make an informed choice, and I encourage you to be adventurous and try all environments.

Private Practice in a Professional Office

Some massage therapists offer their services in a professional office setting, and they do their own scheduling. Similar to a home office but not quite the same, this is one of the more personal settings for receiving massage.

You step away from your own environment and go to the therapist's space instead of having the practitioner come to yours, which helps to relieve you of any responsibilities and potential interruptions before you enter the environment in which to receive your massage. Driving to and from your massage setting may also help you to transition between activities, giving you time to unwind before you lie down on the massage table and before you return to your own life schedule after your appointment. When you arrive for your massage, the scene and mood are already set, and a sanctuary of peace and tranquility greets you.

Private Practice in a Home Office

If you prefer a homier environment than professional offices, try a home office setting. Home office environments vary greatly depending on the lifestyles of massage therapists. Some live alone, some with family, while others live with roommates or pets, and their locations may be rural or urban. The massage room may be in the dwelling or kept separate from it, but all these factors contribute to the environment in which you will receive your massage.

Here, too, you free your life from commitments as you transition and unwind before and after your appointment, while your experience of the massage takes place in a calm and soothing environment.

Outcalls

You may prefer to leave the commute to the therapist and receive your massage in the familiarity and convenience of your own home or hotel room. This is known as an outcall; and a commuting fee, which varies among therapists, is added to the cost of the massage. Considerations for determining an outcall fee are as follows:

1. Packing and transporting the table, sheets, oils, music, and other supplies.
2. Setting up the massage table and support items.

3. Breaking down the table, packing, and transporting the table and supplies.
4. Resetting the table and supplies in the original setting.
5. Mileage and time spent to and from the outcall.

Before the therapist arrives, it is helpful if you prepare a room large enough for the massage table, with extra space beyond the table for the therapist to work around it. The room should be warm or cool enough, with working electric outlets nearby.

If members of the household will be in the environment during your massage, assure your privacy and freedom from responsibilities and interruptions with them beforehand. This is crucial to your relaxing and deriving all the benefits from your massage.

Receiving massage in your own home works well if you can carve out a conducive space and if you are able to set boundaries from the usual home routine.

On-Site Chair Massage

For a lesser commitment to time and money, massage chairs are designed for easy transport to locations such as offices, hair salons, health spas, health-related stores, workshops, conventions, wellness functions, swap meets, farmers' markets, shopping malls, airports, and your home. Similar to outcall massages, the therapist comes to you instead of you having to visit the therapist's space. Additionally, it is an opportunity to combine a massage with an activity you are already doing, such as shopping, keeping a salon appointment, or waiting for your flight when traveling.

The recipient remains clothed and seated in the massage chair, and this enables the therapist to massage head, neck, back, arms, and hands. Many positive benefits are possible in just a short time, and a starting price for a chair massage is generally one dollar per minute.

Cruises and Resorts

Cruises, resorts, and massage encourage time out equally, because if you do not find time in your routine schedule for massage, you have the time now.

Massage therapists work on cruise ships and on the premises of vacation resorts, and they are available many hours of the day. Management will have done its part to find and evaluate a reputable therapist for your benefit, and all you need to do is book your appointment. Receiving a massage earlier in your stay allows you to relax sooner and get the most from your vacation; an early appointment also gives you the best chance for a convenient opening in the therapist's schedule.

Health Spas

Some health spas offer massage with a reduced rate for spa members, and the massage can be used as a reward or incentive for your workouts. Regular massage with fitness workouts decreases muscle soreness and recovery time, thereby increasing your body's performance; massage also lessens and deters potential injuries that may come from a hard workout. Fitness workouts and massage are a natural combination, just as chiropractic and massage go well together. An added advantage is receiving both your fitness workout and massage in one stop.

Day Spas

Day spas provide locally what cruises and resorts offer vacationers, and you receive your massage and spa treatments without having to go away. In these one-stop venues, you can enjoy body wraps that detoxify and rejuvenate, steam showers, saunas, and Jacuzzis; even facial, hair, and nail services may be available.

Student Clinics

Massage schools establish and maintain student clinics for learners requiring completion of their certification criteria. Students working at these clinics have finished the majority of their studies and need a certain number of experiential hours outside their classrooms, and they depend on the experience and knowledge gained from their work in these clinics; therefore, your honest and tactful feedback is of great value. Most students are capable of giving a good massage at this stage of their training, and the benefit to you is the massage fee, which is less than most professional rates because the students are still in training and not yet licensed.

The Chiropractor's Office

Massage and chiropractic have a natural working relationship because muscles move the skeleton, and without them, the skeleton would be a heap of bones on the floor. Tight muscles make it difficult for chiropractors to fine-tune the skeleton and make it hold an adjustment, and this is because tight muscles tend to pull the skeleton back out of alignment. Furthermore, soreness after an adjustment is more likely when muscles are restricted and unyielding, so it is helpful and desirable to receive a massage before a skeletal adjustment, as the massage relaxes muscles and releases the tension that they hold. The bones can then move with greater ease as they are being adjusted by the chiropractor, and they maintain their adjustment better. For this reason, many chiropractors' offices have massage therapists on staff.

Additionally, some insurance companies cover a particular quota of massages per year. Accident-related adjustments cover massage for a particular period and dollar amount, *as long as the patient follows the criteria for frequency and duration of treatment, which is issued by the insurance company.* When massage is given on the premises of the recommended chiropractor, insurance is more likely to cover the cost of the session. Check with your insurance company before receiving your massage, as it may be covered in your policy; but if massage is not a service that your insurance policy covers, do not miss out on treating yourself to one. You are worth it.

Airports

Airports are additional environments in which to receive massage, particularly if you find it challenging to make time for one. Although chair massage opportunities may be found scattered at various airports by individual massage therapists, Massage Bar can seat up to thirteen massage customers at one time in the format of a bar, a unique presentation style that includes 15- and 30-minute massage sessions without the necessity of appointments. Massage Bar established itself as an innovative company in 1993, serving eleven airport locations in the US, and the list is growing. You can learn more at www.massagebar.com.

Make your waiting time before a flight departure an opportunity to receive a massage. You may have been sitting for long periods, sleeping in uncomfortable situations, and changing time zones, but these are perfect reasons to treat yourself to a massage in an effort to counteract the effects of traveling. Even fifteen minutes—the general period for a chair massage—can de-stress a weary or anxious traveler.

≈

As you can see, there are several environments to choose from if you desire a massage. In addition to massage, many establishments sell products such as lotions, creams, eye and neck pillows, essential oils, salts, facial products, and more. However, purchasing these products immediately following your massage and while you are in a relaxed and altered state, may lead to second thoughts later; so before you make decisions that require more thought, allow yourself some time to transition slowly and fully after your massage.

Hospitals

Some progressive hospitals have Integrative Medicine departments that combine conventional medicine and CAM (Complementary and Alternative Medicine), which include services such as Acupuncture, Energy Therapy (Reiki, Therapeutic Touch, Quantum Healing), Hypnosis, Lymphatic Therapy, Therapeutic Massage, CranioSacral Therapy, Reflexology, Meditation, and other relaxation techniques. Practitioners in their field of expertise offer CAM to the community in the form of individual sessions, evening programs, and workshops. Additionally, trained and compassionate volunteers offer meditation, hand massage, reflexology, and other relaxing modalities at the bedside of surgically- and terminally-ill patients.

Points worth rubbing in:
1. Get a massage; it feels so good and does wonders for you. Massage therapists are everywhere.
2. Treat yourself to a massage.
3. Save decisions for later when they require more thought and when you are no longer in an altered, relaxed state.

Chapter 3:
Interviewing the Massage Therapist

A therapist or therapeutic establishment interested in building a rapport with potential clients will answer your massage-related questions on the phone. I have provided the following questions as guidelines to help you find the best therapist for your needs:

1. What type of massage does a therapist perform?

The therapist's repertoire will help you define your needs and facilitate a good match for you. Before you talk to a massage therapist, however, it may be useful to read Chapter 4: Most Common Types of Massage/Bodywork (Techniques, Benefits, and Cautions), which will shape the nature of your questions meant for the therapist.

2. What environment does a therapist work in?

Knowing what to expect about the therapist's environment will help you match your expectations. You may want to revisit Chapter 2: Massage Environments, as there are many options that will suit your needs. Of course, you may want to try several environments if you are not sure what you want, as each has something unique to offer.

3. Where did the therapist train, and how long has he or she been practicing massage?

As yet, no minimum education standard exists for massage therapists; however, according to AMTA's 2011 Massage Therapy Industry Fact Sheet, the number of massage schools and programs in the United States exceeds 300, totaling almost "90,000 nationally certified massage therapists and bodyworkers." Furthermore, the survey states that, to earn national certification, "a massage therapist must demonstrate mastery of core skills and knowledge, pass an exam, uphold the standards of practice and core of ethics of the National Certification Board for Therapeutic Massage & Bodywork, and take part in continuing education." Massage therapists are expected to average an initial training quota of 660 hours.

While a therapist's training is important, it can never surpass experience, which you should consider in your searches. There is much to be gained from a therapist's experience, as it contributes to the practitioner's level of expertise and can affect the outcome of your session. That said, some therapists who are new to the profession are naturals and quite adept at what they do. If you do not have a special need or focus for your massage, do not let training or experience *alone* rule your decision for choosing a therapist. Trust and rapport are primary elements for seeking and receiving massage.

4. What is the therapist's hourly and weekly work schedule?

A compatibility of schedules is also important to your receiving a massage. Apart from the therapist's availability, your considerations for having a massage may be based on several factors involving you and your family, and may include the babysitter's availability, your lunch hours, low traffic times, receiving massage on a day off, and other possibilities.

You might want to also reconsider carrying out those responsibilities and activities that could have an impact on you before and after a massage, so schedule your appointment appropriately while working it into the therapist's schedule. For instance, you would not want to undo the benefits of a massage you have just received by doing any of the following: going straight to the gym for a workout (relaxed muscles are not up to the task of performing strenuous fitness workouts and could risk injury), going grocery shopping, or by engaging in similar physical errands. Post-massage activities may cause you to miss the subtle and rich internal messages resulting from your massage; and because our priorities have a way of shifting in this relaxed, internal massage state, make sure to schedule your appointment wisely, and *invest in your investment.*

5. Where is the therapist located? Why location matters.

A therapist's location is an important consideration when scheduling your appointment. Not only does distance involve travel time and gas money, but it can be a large deterrent after a massage when you are relaxed; most likely, other drivers on the road will not be as calm as you will be following your appointment. Tasks that require your alertness or that demand your sense of responsibility after a massage can undo the benefits you have just acquired, so keep these considerations in mind as you choose a therapist's location to have your massage.

6. What is a therapist's fee? Do therapists give discounts or use a sliding scale?

As a result of several variables such as a therapist's expertise, training, type of massage and establishment, and geographical area, massage fees vary widely and range from $40.00 to $100.00 or more for a one-hour session. You might pay the lower end of the range at student clinics, for practitioners just beginning their careers, and when applying discounts; you will pay the higher end of the range at spas and with types of massage that require more expertise, such as lymphatic massage or craniosacral therapy. Furthermore, the operating costs vary with each situation, and will play a role in the fees therapists charge and any discounts they may offer. While some therapists use an introductory rate for first-time clients, they will also give discounts to students, seniors, and families. In addition, package discounts may be available for clients who are willing to pay in advance for a series of massages. While a sliding scale—variable fees appropriate to different income levels—is not always advertised, the therapist you choose may offer it, so ask if any of these options are available.

Points worth rubbing in:
1. Ask for what you want in a massage.
2. Obtain the best match between you and a therapist.
3. Try more than one therapist for comparison.
4. Choose your time and the therapist's location wisely.

Chapter 4:

Most Common Types of Massage/Bodywork (Techniques, Benefits, and Cautions)

D oes not knowing what to ask for or not knowing what to expect become an obstacle to your receiving massage? This is the case for most people who have never experienced a massage before. Do images of massage in the media—karate chops delivered on boxers in locker rooms, or hands smoothed lightly over a bare back—deter you from receiving a massage, because it looks as though it will hurt or will not be effective or deep enough?

Your unfamiliarity about massage need not keep you from receiving and enjoying its benefits. This chapter covers the most common types of massage, in which I address the following:

Techniques: What manner of touch you can expect from your therapist.

Benefits: The purpose of different massage types and their expected results.

Cautions: Health concerns contrary to receiving some types of massage.

≈

Techniques. You need not choose just one kind of massage, as you can combine several methods of bodywork in a session; but be sure that, before scheduling a particular combination, the types of massage you choose are indeed part of your therapist's repertoire of techniques.

Even if you are less knowledgeable about different massage types, your massage therapist can meet your needs with input from you about your current situation; describe your particular focus for the massage and the outcome that you desire. For instance, you may have a headache, allergies, menstrual cramps, or shoulder and arm tension from long hours at the computer. You may have back pain from routinely carrying a child, a forthcoming exam, divorce, wedding, or important decision that is making you anxious. A medical practitioner or psychologist may have referred you for specific reasons. On the other hand, you may simply want to relax. Naturally, knowing what you need will determine the appropriate method of massage.

Just ahead are a few popular massages, with a brief description about each to get you started. Not all techniques work directly with the skin, and, therefore, would not require your being undressed to receive the work, particularly if nakedness may deter you from receiving massage altogether. Some techniques are shared between different massage types; likewise, some of the benefits are similar. In general, most types of massage release muscle tension, resulting in relaxation and ease of movement. Deep relaxation results in deep breathing and healing, which affect the body, mind, emotions, and spirit; deep breathing increases oxygen to all cells of the body and improves the cardiopulmonary system. Consequently, your massage restores your body with calm, energy, and a sense of overall well-being.

≈

Benefits. Lastly and, perhaps, most importantly, *the benefits of touch alone are significant and vast*. Ashley Montagu explains this so well in his book *Touching: The Human Significance of the Skin* when he says: "Though it may vary structurally and functionally with age, touch remains a constant, the foundation upon which all other senses are based. The skin is the largest sensory organ of the body, and the tactile system is the earliest sensory system to become functional in all species thus far studied—human, animal, and bird" (Montagu 1986, 4–5). Furthermore, Montagu adds, "The central nervous system, which has a principal function keeping the organism informed of what is going on outside it, develops as the inturned portion of the general surface of the embryonic body. The rest of the surface covering, after the differentiation of the brain, spinal cord, and all the other parts of the central nervous system, becomes the skin and its derivatives—hair, nails, and teeth. The nervous system is, then, a buried part of the skin, or alternatively the skin may be regarded as an exposed portion of the nervous system." As you can see, regardless of the type of massage you receive, the benefits of touch alone, and your therapist's quality of touch and presence with you, are immense.

≈

Cautions. Inform your massage therapist of any of the following conditions that you may be experiencing, as certain techniques may have adverse effects for particular situations. Be assured, however, that there *is* a type of massage to suit your need, and you will not have to miss an opportunity to receive one.

Here then are conditions to be cautious of and to inform your therapist about beforehand: heart related conditions such as thrombosis, phlebitis, edema, high blood pressure, and varicose veins; fever, infections, contagious diseases, cancer, and pregnancy; osteoporosis, disk or skeletal problems, joint replacements, arthritis, swelling, fractures, and bruising. Gentler massage modalities such as Craniosacral therapy, Reiki, and other energy systems are recommended for contraindicated conditions (any of the above-mentioned health concerns being contrary to your receiving certain massage types).

For in-depth information and to learn more about the wider range of massage, refer to the book by Thomas Claire titled *Body Work: What Type of Massage to Get And How to Make the Most of It,* published by Basic Health Publications (www.basichealthpub.com). You may also refer to the Selected Bibliography at the end of my book.

Swedish or Circulatory Massage

The terms Swedish and Circulatory are used interchangeably for this massage, which is one of the most popular techniques, and it is often given the first time.

With this type of massage, oils and lotions help to deliver a variety of strokes and pressures for your body, head, and face. Some strokes are long and continuous, defining the whole muscle in a broad sense; other techniques are specific for working out knotted muscles. Kneading, stroking, and tapping with desirable pressure also promote these beneficial effects.

Swedish massage increases circulation and red blood cells, and it helps to break up lactic and uric acid (both toxins) that get trapped in tight muscles; additionally, this technique relieves muscle spasms and overall tension. Swedish massage heightens awareness of your body in general and is best for reducing and relaxing full-body stress. Light to moderate pressure is used.

Pregnancy Massage

Special training is required for the pregnancy massage therapist. If you are receiving any type of massage and are pregnant or if you think you may be pregnant, inform your therapist, as some techniques are not recommended. Extra pillows, bolsters, even body support systems specific for carrying extra weight in breasts and in the abdomen are used while you lay on the massage table. Massage techniques and body positioning (including lying on your side) vary according to each trimester. In the latter trimester, circulatory massage is best because the therapist's touch is light to medium, placing emphasis on the relaxation of muscles, which are tense from carrying mother and fetus. This approach also increases the circulation (as does exercise), and it oxygenates all cells in the body, providing richer nourishment for mother and fetus. This is an added benefit for women who are unable to exercise during pregnancy.

Since drugs are not involved, massage during pregnancy is a healthy option for sciatica, and muscle and joint discomfort. Likewise, relief for symptoms of headaches, congestion, and allergies is possible without the use of drugs; acupressure and massage are applied to the face and head.

Emotional and physical nurturing through massage is even more important during pregnancy, as the link between mother and fetus is strongest at this time, both physically as well as emotionally. The fetus will reflect a calmer, happier, and well-cared-for mother.

Sports Massage

Some massage techniques are similar to isometric exercises (stretching and contracting muscles simultaneously), and these techniques require participation from an active—not passive—recipient to match the therapist's pressure. When a muscle works against the extra load of the therapist's pressure, this work helps the muscle surrender its tension, which it was unable to do on its own. Sports massage works well for muscles that remain tight habitually and that are put through a more strenuous work habit. In addition, this massage can be given to a clothed or naked recipient, and it allows other techniques to be performed without the help of the recipient, such as friction across the fibers of the tendons and ligaments.

Sports massage has two phases: pre-event and post-event. Before an event, the focus is on loosening the ligaments and tendons, as these are most susceptible to injury. The muscles themselves are not massaged before an event, because they would be too relaxed to perform the sports activity. In contrast, post-event massage relaxes the muscles and works out knots that trap lactic acid and uric acid produced by exertion; the result to the massage recipient is less soreness and tightness, and a quicker recovery time which aids the athlete in returning to training workouts sooner and with better performance.

While oil is optional for sports massage, depending on which techniques are used, muscle liniments and products of the same kind may also be applied.

Deep Tissue Massage

With deep tissue massage, pressure in a specific or general area is delivered with sensitivity by the trained therapist's fingers, palms, soft fists, forearms, and elbows; and this technique does not need to be painful to be effective or satisfying to the recipient. To release tension in the body's tissues, the therapist rubs in small amounts of lotion to maintain pressure and depth without pulling the skin or slipping. I like to compare deep tissue massage to sculpting with clay: first, you must knead and warm the clay until it is pliable, and then you can shape it.

Deep tissue massage gains access to deeper layers of tension that muscles hold for long periods; this massage also assists new injuries or symptoms of muscle spasm, limited range of movement, and muscle ache and pain. Relieving tension from tight muscles frees the skeleton, enabling it to move more effortlessly, purposefully, and with a wider range of motion.

In addition, deep tissue massage is beneficial where physical therapy stops. Quite often, prescriptions administered for physical therapy limit the treatment for a set duration, perhaps, one to three sessions a week for six weeks; but when the physical therapy stops, more help may still be needed, and deep tissue massage is appropriate in this case.

Quite often, recipients of deep tissue massage will also seek this treatment for accessing and releasing their emotions. Muscle tension, also called *body armor*, is a term used by therapists to describe tense muscles; and this armor serves as an illusory protection, whereby, the restricted and holding tissue disallows feelings to flow in or find their way out. However, when the armor softens, any withheld emotions will generally become released too, proving that the body-mind connection is very evident in this way.

Shiatsu

Shiatsu (she-ät-sü) is a traditional Japanese healing system which uses light, medium, and firm pressure delivered with the therapist's thumbs, knuckles, palms, elbows, knees, and feet along meridians—energy lines that run along the muscles as pathways. In the Shiatsu system, each muscle group correlates with specific organs. By applying pressure to specific points located on the muscles, the therapist helps release tension from the distressed muscle and restores balance to the individual organs associated with it. For instance, the therapist working the lung meridian would be pressing points along your forearm, between your elbow and wrist. What's more, if an organ is out of balance in any way, the muscle group related to the organ may be tender or weak; by releasing the tension from tender areas, the therapist restores balance to the organ, and the muscle is relieved of tension and discomfort.

Foot Reflexology

Foot reflexology is suitable for the majority of people and situations, and it is desirable for those with modesty or touch concerns. The feet are the focus of this massage technique, although this type of Reflexology can be integrated easily with full-body massage. Pressure is applied and sustained to points along the bottoms, tops, and sides of both feet, and this pressure stimulates reflexes through nerve endings in the foot. Each reflex point relates to a particular body part and vital organ; and as these reflex points are worked on and as release occurs, balance is restored to the related areas of the body. The entire body is addressed through the feet, and the recipient often feels as though he or she has had a full body massage.

Foot reflexology is especially good for diabetics because it increases circulation in the feet. It is also beneficial for bringing awareness and grounding to the feet for balance and coordination, so when the feet are relaxed and open to receiving the weight of the body, the entire posture is affected positively.

Reiki

Reiki (ray-key) is a Japanese term, meaning universal life energy; this same life force is within and around all living beings, and it nourishes us and keeps us alive.

When receiving a Reiki session, the recipient is fully clothed and the practitioner's hands rest lightly on or above the recipient. Reiki works with the energy field that surrounds the body and that is linked to the physical body through the connection between the body's chakras and the endocrine glands. Chakras are non-physical, spiraling energy wheels located along the spine, and all seven chakras correlate with the body's physical organs and their associated emotions. The crown chakra is the seventh chakra, which resides energetically at the top of the head; this chakra connects us with our spiritual self and is correlated to the endocrine system. Hence, Reiki's gentle method affects the body's physical, emotional, mental, and spiritual aspects. Furthermore, Reiki can be used alone or combined with other massage systems.

Recipients of Reiki commonly experience states of deep calmness in their sessions because of the sixth chakra's relation to the nervous system. Some people relax so deeply (as if asleep), but their calmness offers a different awareness, as though they have been transported far away and are very peaceful. Recipients may feel the Reiki energy at work during a session, while others report that they do not feel anything until after the session, whereas some recipients experience nothing at all. When recipients *do* feel the energy at work, few see colors, recall incidents from the past, and feel the presence of those who have passed on; still others have felt their skeletons adjust gently, as though through a chiropractic adjustment. Although Reiki's technique is subtle, its results can be profound.

Since pressure is not exerted nor strokes applied to increase circulation, Reiki is beneficial for people with osteoporosis, severe varicose veins, inflammation, fever, and painful conditions such as arthritis and disk problems; Reiki is also good for other conditions, which I have listed at the beginning of this chapter in the section marked "Cautions."

Other energy modalities are Zero Balancing, Touch for Health (Kinesiology), Therapeutic Touch, Jin Shin, and Teller Touch, to name a few.

CranioSacral Therapy (CST)

CST affects the emotions, musculature, skeleton, and connective tissue of the entire body via the central nervous system (CNS). The cranium (skull), and the sacrum (the triangular bone at the base of the spine), are intimately involved with the CNS and are the main areas where this therapy takes place. Through gentle and sensitive touch, the CST practitioner facilitates the release of holding patterns in the body's connective tissue and in the compressed bones of the skull. A few causes of skull bone compression are the birthing process, falls, blows to the head, and day-to-day situations that involve wearing hats, eye glasses, headphones, helmets, and hair accessories too tightly.

This release through CST enables parts of the brain that are restricted by the compression to function as intended. The brain being the message center, CST helps it to communicate with all functions of the body using more clarity and efficiency; and it can be said that CST works in this way from the inside out.

However, CST also works from the outside in, through the skin; but direct skin contact is not necessary, hence the recipient is clothed when receiving this type of therapy. The practitioner uses light pressure or holding to assist an area of tissue with its release or with its need to unwind. In the process, other tissue restrictions are also released because they are all connected through the skin, which encompasses the entire body's surface and its internal makeup. To use a visual metaphor, the result is similar to pulling the end of a large sheet; eventually all creases unfold and move as one. The key to the CST system is the absence of force as well as the practitioner's patience for the release of tissue restrictions in accordance with the timing of the recipient's body.

CST is not considered massage nor is it considered chiropractic, even though the result may be similar; however, CST can be combined with massage or stand on its own. More and more, massage therapists, chiropractors, physical therapists, and other health practitioners are including CST in their repertoire.

Like Reiki and other energy systems, CST is very gentle, which makes it a good choice for those who cannot endure pressure due to osteoporosis, and for those with painful maladies and some conditions not recommended for massage. CST is beneficial in the prevention of Alzheimer's disease, dementia, and nerve disorders, and it is gentle enough for infants, especially when birth trauma is involved.

CranioSacral Therapy was developed by Dr. John Upledger. Other similar modalities developed by Upledger and Jean-Pierre Barral that involve the central nervous system are Core Energetics, Zero Balancing, Healing From the Core, Visceral Manipulation, and more.

≈

As you can see, the power of touch has the potential to affect body, mind, emotion, and spirit, no matter the modality. The type of massage technique (modality) that you choose is just another path to get the care that you need, whereas your openness to the technique and the therapist's quality of touch and presence will help to determine the outcome of your experience.

Massage/Bodywork is appropriate for all ages, from infancy through to the elderly, and it is good for pets too. There are massage classes designed for the lay person; and learning massage for yourself, family, and friends can be well suited for home remedies, nurturing, and finding closeness with one another. For the availability of classes, inquire at massage schools and health food stores, check community bulletin boards and Internet massage sites, or find local practitioners to coach you individually or to give classes to the community.

Summary of the Benefits of Massage/Bodywork

The physical benefits of massage are as follows:
1. It relaxes the body
2. Increases circulation
3. Increases flexibility and range of motion
4. Decreases chronic pain
5. Strengthens the immune system
6. Reduces the effects of stress
7. Improves nerve function

8. Assists in better sleep

9. Improves skin and muscle tone

10. Reduces tension headaches

11. Improves posture and balance

12. Calms the nervous system

13. Lowers blood pressure

14. Reduces heart rate

15. Slows respiration

16. Promotes deeper and more effective breathing

17. Reduces swelling and scarring

18. Increases tissue metabolism

19. Decreases muscular deterioration

20. Relieves cramps and muscle spasms

21. Relieves tired and aching muscles

22. Increases blood and lymph flow

23. Speeds the removal of toxins and metabolic waste

24. Stimulates the release of endorphins

25. Speeds recovery time from workouts, injuries, and illness

26. Increases red blood cell count

27. Loosens tight muscles, tendons, and ligaments

28. Heightens the senses and body-awareness

29. Assists the flow of energy (chi), bringing greater health to vital organs

30. Combines well with—and aids more results with—other modalities such as chiropractic, acupuncture, psychotherapy, physical therapy, and more

The mental and emotional benefits of massage are as follows:

1. Helps you access, release, and understand emotions

2. Restores humor

3. Reduces anxiety
4. Enhances self-esteem and self-image
5. Improves concentration
6. Promotes verbal and creative expression
7. Subdues excessive emotions
8. Promotes the making of healthy choices
9. Provides an overall sense of well being

Certainly, the benefits of massage are abundant. Massage is a natural treatment for infants and children, and it can be helpful for people in difficult situations. For instance, massage can assist the blind, deaf, and mute; comfort the elderly living alone or anyone isolated for any reason; help release past traumas such as those who are physically or sexually abused; and come to the aid of victims of accidents, divorce, and other loss. Massage assures needful recipients like the sickly and aging; it lets them know that someone is there with them through the administering of appropriate and caring touch as a means of communication. When we feel better, others around us feel it too, making us healthier and happier individuals in a healthy society.

Points worth rubbing in:
1. The benefits of touch are immeasurable.
2. All ages benefit from massage.
3. Inform your massage therapist of any cautious conditions.
4. Be assured there is an appropriate type of massage for everyone.
5. Your openness to massage and your therapist helps determine the outcome of your experience.

Chapter 5:
You Want Massage but Cannot Afford It (Ways to Afford Massage)

"I can't afford massage" is a common objection I hear, and I believe it to be one of the largest roadblocks to receiving massage. However, affording massage may be easier than you think, and I explain how in this chapter.

Gift Certificates

The ultimate satisfaction in affording massage is receiving a gift certificate from someone you know. Because we often view massage as a luxury, is there a more appropriate time to ask for a session than a forthcoming holiday or special occasion? Your opportunities to receive gift certificates for massage are plenty: You have Christmas, Valentine's Day, Mother's Day, and Father's Day too; and there are birthdays, weddings, anniversaries, graduations, promotions, marathons, accomplishments of all kinds, and, as always, "just because." A common tendency is to give what we would like to receive. If massage is what you want, ask for one, and if you would like your massage from a specific facility or practitioner, provide your gift giver with the necessary information.

On the other hand, when presenting someone with a massage, be sure the recipient would actually like one. Incomprehensible as it may seem, not everyone likes or wants a massage; consequently, your gift may not be received in the way that you intended, and it could become a source of aggravation between you and the receiver. In some cases, and feeling pressured and guilt ridden, recipients redeem their massage gifts just to ease their burden, and this results in therapists massaging clients who do not want to be there.

Nevertheless, if you do gift someone a massage that you know will be appreciated, emphasize the recipient's notion of luxury and include a personal chauffeur for the session, but only if the enhancement fits your budget and if it feels right. Furthermore, if the chauffeur is also the giver of the gift certificate, he or she will be embraced by the happy vibration and massage-glow of the recipient, knowing without a doubt, how well the gift was received.

Chair Massage

Chair massage, which I discuss in Chapter 2 (Massage Environments), involves the least time and monetary commitment. The general fee is $1.00 per minute, and ten to fifteen minutes is a standard time for receiving a chair massage, but less or more is an option. Massage chairs are designed to sit comfortably and come with a face cradle in which to rest your head; you remain fully clothed, while the therapist massages your head, neck, shoulders, back, arms, and hands.

There are numerous locations to obtain your chair massage, and you can find therapists on site at health food stores, airports, malls, hair salons, corporations, conventions, wellness functions, and more. The list is as long as the possibilities. Many massage therapists own a table and chair and will do chair massage in their practice spaces, so be sure to ask if this service is available.

You can obtain relaxation, rejuvenation, and overall well-being in a fifteen-minute chair massage. One fact to keep in mind when considering a chair massage is that it is often done in public, and this visibility can deter some people from using this option. If this stops you, keep in mind that your inhibitions and surroundings soon fade away, as the benefits of massage begin to overtake your awareness; the experience is similar to moments when you drift into sleep and the external world begins to fall away gradually.

Half-Hour Table Massage

Another way to keep your cost down and retain the quality and expertise of your therapist is to schedule a shorter massage. A thirty-minute massage can get you more than you think, especially if you use the session to focus on specific areas of your body, as opposed to your having a full-body massage. For instance, if your main concern is your neck, shoulders, and back (a concern shared by the majority of the population), your massage therapist will pro-portion time for this request in the allotted half hour. However, if you must also have your feet or any other desired part of your body massaged, the therapist will need to absorb time from your half-hour session for the additional work.

A full body massage in a half hour is possible but not recom-mended, as each part receives very little attention in this short time frame. Therefore, to address the entire body more thoroughly and while staying within the half-hour time frame, have your massage in two segments: in your first week, massage the lower body; in the following week, address the upper body. You and your therapist can experiment session by session with what work's best for you.

Student Clinics

Student clinics charge considerably less than experienced and licensed massage establishments, the obvious reason is that students are acquiring experience while still in training. Furthermore, expertise among students may vary greatly—some students are naturals when it comes to massage and may be very adept early on in their training, whereas others are still honing their skills. As well, some students will discover that massage is not their calling. Should you seek out your massage at a student clinic near you, your tactful and honest feedback is valuable to the students involved and to the future of the massage profession. Student clinics can be found by contacting massage schools in your area; simply check your Yellow Pages, call directory assistance, or conduct an Internet search.

Budgeting

According to the results of the *2009 AMTA Industry Survey*, clients pay an average of $63.00 per one hour of massage. Let us round off this number to $60.00 and divide it by 30, the average number of days in a month; what we get is $2.00 per day. Looking at your daily expenses and spending habits, you can try to cut back on some of these expenses and habits so you can afford your massage.

Does your lifestyle permit you to save $2.00 a day for massage? Perhaps, you eat out every day or frequently. Take lunch for instance—if your average lunch outside costs you $10, and if you were to replace six lunches each month with a homemade sandwich, soup, or salad, you will have budgeted for one monthly massage. So it isn't difficult to budget for a massage when you make up your mind to have one.

Self-Massage

Only you will know *where* your body wants the attention in a massage, how much pressure you would like, and for how long. Let me preface this topic by saying that we have a cultural taboo against touching ourselves. However, children explore their world naturally, using their senses of sound, smell, taste, sight, and touch; their exploration through curiosity and instinct often leads them to knowledge re-discovered as adults. For instance, as a child, I had many ear infections and abscesses, but I discovered that if I pressed the area around my ear, I would get temporary relief. When my parents saw me pushing on my red, painful ear, they told me to stop so I wouldn't make the pain worse; however, I knew that pushing down on my ear helped to ease the pain, but it also scared my parents, so I continued to press the points in private. Much later in massage school, I studied acupressure, and it confirmed what I discovered instinctively as a child.

To get started with self-massage, you might begin by giving yourself a foot massage when listening to the radio, watching television, or riding as a passenger. Maybe you prefer to make the activity less distracting by giving the massage your undivided attention. If so, begin by turning off the phone, turning on some relaxing music, and setting out your favorite lotions and aromas.

Knowledge of technique is not necessary for the natural world of touch. Be child-like, explore, and discover feeling through your senses. Massage your entire foot as though you have never seen or touched it before; learn what your foot likes most and satisfy it some more. Keep tuning in to what it wants and needs, and be generous with this time for yourself, and then continue with other areas of your body in the same way, by exploring and enjoying the process. Foot massage and full body massage are both very transformational to the body and mind.

When you are finished, pause and acknowledge what you are feeling. Massage often leads to a meditative state, and you may drift off into a nap or sleep through the night. If you are continuing with your day, be sure to transition slowly from your massage as you carry the qualities and effects of the massage into the rest of your day; others may respond to you in kind and will benefit from your experience. You may also find that you enjoy people and activities more in this state.

Massage Classes

Perhaps you have been doing massage for yourself and for others, and finding that you like it so much, you would like to learn more. That being so, you may find enthusiasts like yourself who are interested in exchanging massages.

You do not need to commit to a certified program in order to take classes; there are classes available for the lay person not intending to be a professional practitioner. These classes, which can be held in one evening or as weekend workshops, are offered at massage schools and by massage therapists for their clients and for the community. There are three popular classes, namely, couple's massage, foot reflexology, and basics for beginners. You can look into these classes by contacting massage schools and massage therapists in your area, and use the information from these classes for yourself, family, and friends.

Maybe you have been exchanging massage with your spouse, children, siblings, friends, or someone else. You may feel more confident than the other person does, and so you suggest taking a class together—an idea that motivates you both, although you may want to keep an eye out for troublesome situations, as in the example I outline below.

When I taught couple's massage classes, it was common for one partner to approach me in confidence and express gratitude for the fact that I taught the class, because the confiding partner did not feel satisfied with the quality of massage being returned in exchange. At a later point, the other massage partner would also come to me in private and say the very same thing. In the end, we all had a good laugh when I shared the story with my students.

We *can* gain something from learning. Massage classes teach more than technique; they instruct us on the proper use of the body, so neither giver nor receiver will feel uncomfortable during the massage. The classes also impart listening skills that involve asking crucial questions meant to uncover what a recipient wants and how couples can sustain a two-way feedback system. A common approach for couples giving massage is for one individual to give the kind of massage that he or she would like to receive, overlooking the differing requests of the partner. Even so, we need to communicate our differences and respond to them in massage's two-way feedback process.

The proverb "different strokes for different folks" applies literally in the massage setting. In a typical scenario where a husband and wife massage each other, he likes a great deal of pressure when receiving his massage, so *that* is what he gives her, but she complains that it hurts. He then informs his wife that it takes pressure to bring her relief and that his effort will make her feel really good when he is done; but when it is her turn to give him a massage, she proceeds with gentle stroking, very much in the way that she would like to receive hers. He asks for a great deal of pressure, and she explains that the gentleness will relax him all over and that he will not feel so tense afterwards. He insists on more pressure, so she gives all that she has which never seems to be enough for him, even though her hands and arms begin to hurt. At the very least, their exchange ends with frustration and dissatisfaction.

The couple's class may help the female partner find ways to give more pressure without hurting herself. Learning to give someone the kind of massage that he or she asks for and asking for what you want in a massage so that you get it, are both essential ingredients for giving and receiving massage—which can bring closeness and bonding in the home, and among family members and friends.

Bartering

Bartering primarily involves an exchange of skills and services that are as variable as are the parties involved in the exchange. If you do not believe you have something to offer, find out what the other party needs, and, together, you may both agree on something you did not think of earlier. I once received massages in exchange for baking homemade bread! Bartering services can include chiropractic care, auto mechanical work, haircuts, dental work, veterinarian appointments, housecleaning, cooking, yard work, babysitting, payments toward rent, and computer and technology support. The list is as vast as each person's needs and wants.

Some people say bartering works although others disagree, but there is an art to bartering if both parties are to be satisfied. The following savvy tips should help:

1. Be sure the barter offers something you really want, just as you would do when paying cash for a product or service.
2. Declare a value that makes you both feel good. Call around for prices if you are not sure what amount to pay in trade, just as you would do when paying cash.
3. Set a completion date for the barter, as some projects can be long-winded; if this is the case, declare checkpoints along the way.
4. Allow time to think it over. Address any concerns before agreeing to do the trade, and be sure that both parties feel right about it from the beginning.
5. Barter labor for labor; pay cash for materials.
6. Put it in writing and sign it before either service is given.

Do remember that Uncle Sam requests a share, and you can find all the necessary contracts and tax forms from bartering organizations that you decide to approach. Because the barter will be between individuals, be sure both parties have records and receipts of services traded.

Enjoy your massages and your supplemental earning power through bartering.

Discounts

Introductory Rates. Some therapists and establishments give a discount for first time clients, so long as the discount is not combined with a gift certificate or with any other discounts. You may need to ask if discounts are available, because not every therapist or massage establishment advertises them.

≈

Series Discounts. These discounts are given when you buy several massages at one time and pay for the services in advance, whereas the price break is determined by the amount of massages purchased in the series—a set of eight massages, of course, has a bigger discount than that of four. One of my clients bought his wife a package of twelve massages every Christmas, and she enjoyed her one-and-a-half-hour session each month during the year.

≈

Referral Discounts. Some therapists and establishments give a discount to regular and returning clients for each new client they refer. The amount of the discount varies.

≈

Seniors and Students. The therapist or establishment involved in the transaction will set the fee for such discounts; and as a reminder to students, a valid identification may be required.

≈

Sliding Scales. Some therapists offer a sliding scale in the form of a price range, which the client and practitioner or establishment will discuss and determine when scheduling the massage appointment.

Please note that not all therapists will offer discounts, although it does not hurt to ask beforehand.

≈

Medical Insurance. Some medical insurance plans cover a specific amount of massages each year, so be sure to look into your individual plan for details. You may also want to double-check with your medical insurance carrier before assuming that your massage is covered; and if it is covered, make sure to provide your massage therapist with necessary insurance forms and anything else required by your medical plan.

≈

Extension Plans. I discuss extension plans in Chapter 1, which also apply to this section on discounts. Many medical insurance plans now offer a medical extension plan, which is merely a listing of practitioners who have discounted their fees for this purpose. This extension plan is not the same as the services covered by your insurance provider, and the two plans are distinct from one another. The extension plan was developed by insurance companies that do not cover alternative health services such as massage, and the plan works like this: The insurance provider contacts interested massage therapists who agree to discount their fees 10%–25% for insurance plan members. Your insurance provider then suggests a list of participating massage therapists you can call. *However, the only involvement your insurance company has with this transaction is providing you with the names of therapists.* You pay the therapist the discounted fee once you receive your massage. When scheduling your massage, it would be wise to confirm the massage therapist's participation in the extension plan and the affiliated fee that you hope to pay.

Massage Is Your Birthright, Not a Luxury

Sometimes our inner and outer critics will spout remarks about massage with comments like "I feel guilty spending money on myself this way," and "How do you rate getting a massage?" or even "Another massage?" Our voices might also exclaim, "A one-and-a-half-hour massage!" and even ask, "Wow, how often do *you* get a massage?" Indeed, we are more likely to take on an extra job or responsibility and live through our stress than practice self care, which gives us pleasure and relief of stress-related symptoms.

There are numerous reasons for self care in our day-to-day lives; and depriving ourselves of the benefits of massage and delaying its inevitability might even exasperate situations in our bodies that could result in spasm or injury.

We seek permission for self care that is pleasurable through massage, although we may lack the support that makes us feel good. Truth is, it feels good to feel good, and it feels good to be around people who feel good; and until we are on the massage table again, we tend to forget just how good a massage feels.

Allow me to suggest the following reminders that will help you: 1) Keep a journal, or record your experience right off the massage table, 2) Take a before and after photograph of yourself and hang it on your refrigerator door, and 3) Ask someone close to you to remind you just how good you felt after your last massage. So, the next time you are struggling with your inner and outer critics about getting a massage, revisit these reminders.

Life's challenges earn us the right to seek massage; self care and nurturing create compassionate, peaceful people. Furthermore, I believe that massage is your birthright, not a luxury.

Points worth rubbing in:
1. Massage is your birthright.
2. There are many ways to afford massage.
3. Feeling good promotes good health.
4. Self care and nurturing produces compassion and well-being.

≈

Bette's Story.
I arrived at my mid-forties without paying much attention to my body. I pushed it relentlessly, expecting it to do all that I asked of it. It was about this time that my body started talking back to me with a stiff neck and sore knees. Fortunately, I began receiving massages, and during one of the first sessions, I came to a realization: a sense of love and appreciation for my body came over me. My body had endured so much with little complaint and without even receiving a simple "thank you" from me. From that time on, getting a massage was my way of saying "thank you" to my body.

Part Two

SHOWING UP FOR THE MASSAGE: Now that you know who you want and what you want, what do you do when you get there?

Chapter 6:
What the Therapist Should Know about You

Health questionnaires are commonly required for first-time clients, and some therapists collect the information verbally; but as there are many reasons for receiving a massage, it is important for your therapist to know what you want from your session and if you have any injuries, illnesses, or conditions, because this helps to customize the appropriate session for you.

For instance, osteoporosis, disk or skeletal problems, high blood pressure, medications, pregnancy, joint replacements, arthritis, and cancer are all considerations for the type of massage you will receive. There are techniques your therapist would and would not use because of these, and other, conditions, so it is important to inform her.

Your wants may vary from session to session; they may simply be your need to relax or to understand how you accumulate your tension, prompting you to learn what you can do between massages to lessen your stress. You can use massage concurrently with physical therapy treatments or when physical therapy concludes; and because physical therapy works the affected area only, massage can address the rest of the body as well. You may be immobile or convalescing from surgery, or you may have an injury and be unable to exercise; in that case, massage is a good replacement for exercise, because massage milks and kneads the muscles in a way that is similar to exercise. Muscle spasms, sinus problems, headaches, and menstrual cramps are all worthy of massage, as are chronic tensions from an old injury or acute symptoms from a current situation. Referring health professionals such as psychologists and physicians also recommend massage to reinforce or round out the work you are doing with them. Consequently, the more you communicate your needs, the better a therapist can address them.

Points worth rubbing in:
1. Massage can help many physical situations, or it can just relax you. Ask for what you want and need.
2. Be informed of contraindications, and inform your therapist about them.
3. When appropriate, combine massage with other health modalities.

Chapter 7:
Meeting Your Needs before Massage

The ideal way to receive a massage is with *you* being your only focus. Any distraction that interrupts this focus can affect your ability to receive the full potential of your massage. Therefore, it is best to take care of your business and personal needs before arriving for your session; doing so will give you a quality break, making you unavailable to anyone or any situation for at least one hour and more.

Communications

Cell phones and pagers have become like human appendages, so that we depend on them completely; when left on during massages, these devices can startle relaxed clients and disrupt the concentration of massage therapists. I highly recommend that you turn off your cell phone or pager; and, beforehand, inform those depending on you that you will be unavailable. When you take quality time out for yourself and remain free of responsibilities for an hour, you can return to those who depend on you with more clarity and energy. When they also experience the benefits of your massages, they will want to do their part to support you.

Food Needs

Hunger can be a distraction from your massage, and it is difficult to relax your body when hunger pains call you away; but massage can also be uncomfortable if you receive it with a full stomach, so it is best to eat lightly before your session. For some people, hunger may also mean blood sugar imbalances, and these imbalances not only affect the physical body with lethargy or angst, but they also affect the emotions. Anxiety, sadness, and anger are among many of the emotions. If you are receiving massage specifically for emotional release, you would not want to confuse fleeting emotions caused by blood sugar with your deep seated emotions; therefore, centering and stabilizing your body by satisfying its nutritional needs will allow you more self awareness, clarity, and relaxation during your massage.

Water Intake and Outflow

A full bladder can also be very distracting to a massage. You may lie on the massage table thinking that you can make it to the end of the session without having to excuse yourself; however, if you must visit the bathroom, you will find yourself begrudgingly attired in minimum clothing or wrapped in a toga-style sheet.

Some therapists try to make their clients' bathroom visits more convenient by offering smocks for quick and easy use, although some clients would rather wear their own clothes than be seen in smocks.

You will most likely want to avoid such interruptions by drinking small amounts of liquids before your massage or by emptying your bladder beforehand.

Allowing Enough Time to Get There

The following is a common pre-massage scenario: You hurry and get as much done as you possibly can before leaving for your massage. You check your watch frequently and squeeze in a few errands, including a little shopping; then you check your watch again because three people have lined up at the store's cash register when you approach it. You take note of how many items they have to ring up, and you estimate how much time that might take; your stress, however, is accumulating whether you notice it or not.

You know you were already pushing the clock when you went on your errands. Now you feel your muscles contract between your shoulder blades while you wait impatiently, and your breath shortens with every minute delayed and with the possibility that this delay will make you late.

When it is your turn, you pay, take your receipt and purchase, and drop your change in your pocket as you hurry to your car. Your arms and shoulders tense up while you drive fast and stay alert, but you're going faster than the other cars, faster still to gain back the time you lost while waiting in the unexpected line back at the store.

Your stress rises while you look for a parking space; there are fewer than usual, although you find one at the far end of the lot.

You park then walk briskly through the office building, checking your watch and feeling your stomach muscles tighten because you are late—you've been late before. You slow down when you notice how conspicuously fast you are walking in the unhurried and quiet massage environment.

Taking a deep breath, you anticipate your therapist's irritation for your being late. You greet her briefly and get onto the table, arriving just past your appointed time; but your muscles tighten even more as your therapist enters the room, folds back the sheet, and places her hands on your back, although her hands feel a bit tense to you—or is it your back that's tense? Perhaps, the tightness you experience is just your conscience hounding you.

Regardless, you accumulated considerable tension in this scenario and lost your full massage time, as the massage therapist must remain prompt and professional for the next client. Unfortunately, you have deprived yourself of the relaxation you wanted.

≈

In contrast, I recommend the following scenario: Allow ample time to get to your massage appointment and put aside any last-minute errands. Drive safely while you cruise in the slow or right lanes, and listen to your favorite radio station or a selected piece of music. Enjoy the scenery, notice the subtle changes in the sky's colors, revel in each moment, and arrive earlier than your appointed time, perhaps, fifteen minutes ahead.

When you enter the waiting room, feel the shift in energy as you close the front door and the world behind you. Bask in the quiet, the peace, and the serenity of the low-lit and gentle atmosphere, with pleasing aromas that waft in from a massage room only a few short steps away. Sip some pure filtered water, wrap a warm rice sock around your neck, and begin relaxing (I show you how to make a rice sock below). Close your eyes, slip off your shoes and notice your breath slowing and deepening, your weight becoming heavier in the chair, and the chair rising up to meet your weight. Indulge in a deeper breath, follow it with a satisfying sigh, and then savor the stillness that follows before your body takes its next long and luxurious inhalation.

You hear a slight click when the door opens slowly and gentle music enters the waiting room. Open your eyes and you see your massage therapist engulfed in the aura of the massage she has just completed; you nod and exchange a silent greeting, knowing that the best for you is yet to come.

≈

So fifteen more minutes gained with no errands, and this is all it takes for you to experience the second scenario I play out here instead of the first. After all, your happiness is a matter of creating what you are willing to create. Furthermore, you can apply the second scenario to other appointments and activities as well, and your choice can be the start of a new lifestyle with self-nurturing, massage, and less stress.

Points worth rubbing in:
1. Prepare in advance for your quality time out.
2. Arrive unhurried, allowing time to transition and relax before your massage.
3. The less knots and stress you bring to the massage, the more you have to gain.
4. Apply what you learn from your massages and enjoy them as your lifestyle changes.

≈

The Rice Sock: To create one of your very own, all you need is two and one-half pounds of uncooked rice and two over-the-calf men's tube socks, size 10–15. Put the rice in one sock and tie a knot at the end of it. Slip the second sock over the rice-filled sock, as a pillow case that you can launder.

To use your new rice sock, microwave it for two to three minutes, place it around your neck and shoulders or on any other beckoning area. Relax beneath the gentle weight and enjoy the moist heat. Share this nurturing aid with family and friends in your home.

Caution: Do not sleep with the rice sock on your neck, as the heaviness may lessen blood flow; and *do* let it air out after use. As well, do not put the sock away while it is still moist with heat because the rice will mildew.

Rice socks, hot tea, literature, aroma, and music— all greetings of relaxation—vary among massage establishments.

Chapter 8:

What to Wear (Before, During, and After)

Keep it simple. Arrive in clothes that you plan on wearing for the day, or bring a change of clothing. To receive your massage, you can opt to be naked, keep your underwear on, or wear a swim suit or trunks; if you choose to be fully clothed during your massage, wear something comfortable and loose like sweat pants and a top. Loose clothing assists the therapist in kneading and coaxing tight muscles, more so than clothing with pockets, seams, belts, zippers, buttons, collars, cuffs, and tight fabrics that corset and imprint your body. Honoring your modesty level is important, as it assists in your trusting the therapist and opening up to the massage.

Take advantage of an environment without pretenses. Just as you expect to see makeup, hair, and attire that are appropriate for a business setting, massage therapists expect to see their clients arrive in relaxed clothing and leave undaunted by their post-massage appearance, even when it includes hair that is tousled after a good scalp massage. What a relief this can be!

One of my clients had this process perfected. She got off the table after her massage, threw on two garments of clothing, stuffed her underwear in her pockets, and did not bother to smooth out the hair at the nape of her neck where the massage oil caused her hair to turn upward. Then she left to teach her Aikido class in her blissful and unpretentious state. (If you need the therapist to be careful with your hair, make your intention clear, and the practitioner will know to accommodate that request.)

Massage is like the metamorphosis of a caterpillar into a butterfly, because it frees you from limiting influences such as the density of the body's tension, and obsessive-compulsive thoughts and emotions. Moreover, massage offers a renewed perspective on your wellbeing and purpose. Should you prefer, bring a fresh change of clothing to match the way you feel in this new state, or simply stay the way you are, particularly if your schedule takes you back to work or to another event.

If you live in a cooler climate, extra clothing for warmth is highly recommended after your massage. While lying sedentary on the table, your body temperature drops as it does at night when you sleep, so you will want to maintain your new relaxed state by dressing warmly. If you are cold, your muscles will tense up again, undoing some of what you gained, and you do not want to let this happen.

How Much to Undress (True Men's Stories)

A massage therapist and I once provided a simultaneous outcall for two couples, and all four massages were to be given in a home that belonged to one of the couples. The wives had arranged for us to administer the massages first, following which the group would have wine and sushi as a fun way for close friends to spend an evening together.

The men had never received massages before; the women had, however, and they volunteered to receive their massages first while their male partners waited their turns. The men talked and talked, and they eventually consumed two bottles of wine while anticipating their turns with a fair amount of anxiousness.

When the women finished their massages, they went on to enjoy some wine, too, and they talked and relaxed while their partners took their turns on the massage tables; but the women were also surprised at how much wine the men had consumed, and asked their partners why they drank so much.

This is when we all learned of the men's anxieties about receiving massage for the first time, which they revealed in comic-relief style. One of the men said that his wife told him he would need to strip down, and he was very apprehensive about the suggestion. All the same, he did not realize how pleasurable the massage would be. Had he known beforehand, he would have focused on the pleasure and not on his apprehension; he also said he did not think it necessary to take his underwear off to enjoy the massage, and that he would have been more comfortable progressing toward *that* with future sessions.

The other man had a different perspective, however. He was not told anything beforehand and did not know what to expect, and he was uncomfortable because he did not wish to be presumptuous. He had a vision of the therapist saying, "Oh, my God, you took all your clothes off! What do you think this is?" He also believed that "most men are regarded as dogs," and he was scared to death of being labeled the same, thereby projecting an expectation of something—some oddity—unrelated to massage. Of course, most of his concerns were centered around what others thought of him, and he even wondered if we, his massage therapists, thought they were strange for having a little party with wine and sushi following their massage sessions. Had we also wondered what they might be doing after we leave? He was curious to learn the truth to the end.

Looking ahead, he said he would like to know what to expect before getting on the table, including details about leaving his underwear on or taking it off. Being shy and uncomfortable, the man was not about to ask the therapist these questions and preferred that she take the initiative.

≈

Being a professional massage therapist, I appreciated the candidness and willingness of these two men to disclose issues that were uncomfortable for them; and in response to what we therapists might think of them, I could counter with the same. Negative connotations are often associated with massage, with a few resting on the dark side. Even so, both the therapist and client want assurance of a safe and trustworthy environment, so *draping* is one aspect for reassurance, which I discuss next.

In conclusion, I would like to add that these direct and personal stories were disclosed after the massage sessions, and I have permission from the two men to relate their experiences in my own words.

Draping

If you are unclothed for the type of massage you are receiving, you will be lying between two sheets throughout the massage. The top sheet is called a drape and is required by law in most states. The online code of ethics for the National Certification Board for Therapeutic Massage & Bodywork (NCBTMB) requires practitioners to follow this procedure: "Provide draping and treatment in a way that ensures the safety, comfort and privacy of the client" (NCBTMB 2008, under part XII of the "Code of Ethics"). With draping, the part of the body being massaged will be the only area that remains undraped. For instance, the therapist will uncover your leg from under the drape, massage your leg, and then re-drape it; she will then do the same with each part of your body she massages. If the client is female, the therapist will drape the client's breasts while massaging her abdomen; and at no time are breasts or the pubic area for both genders exposed during massage.

Nakedness and Vulnerability

Nudity during massage can raise uncomfortable feelings for other reasons, and many people have disclosed to me that *this* is the reason they have delayed receiving their first massage.

Nakedness and touch are often associated with sexuality, and we have learned to experience such intimate contact only with a partner; however, receiving massage routinely will lessen the association of sex with touch and replace sexual tension with relaxation.

Other associations of nakedness may be made with relation to doctors' offices, hospitals, and locker rooms in schools, for example. Nudity may bring up body-shame messages instilled in us by our parents, siblings, peers, and society; and it can affect victims of sexual abuse and those raised in families where nakedness was permitted only in private quarters. For these very reasons, the massage environment is an opportunity to heal residual feelings from these incidents, because you can inform the therapist of any negative "touch issues" which reside in your past. By receiving appropriate touch through massage, you gain a new and positive association with close physical contact, and you are also presented with an opportunity to verbalize your feelings of past incidents and current ones. Furthermore, if you are uncomfortable with anything your therapist does during your massage, then say so! An example of this may be if the therapist undrapes your buttocks to work on your gluteal muscles, or if the therapist gets up on the table to work on you with more pressure or leverage, which would be appropriate to the setting *only if the client's trust and comfort (yours) is there through it all*. You may end the massage at any point should your discomfort increase and you do not get the response you want, if you do not feel safe at any time, or if you do not find it safe to communicate your needs.

Honor Your Modesty Level

It is important to honor your modesty level, because if you are uncomfortable in any way, you will react to your massage with more tension and less receptivity, and this opposition will keep you from receiving the benefits of massage and the good feelings associated with it.

The amount of clothing you leave on, however, is entirely up to you; and you can still receive a satisfying massage if you leave all your clothes on. Your therapist will customize your massage accordingly.

Points worth rubbing in:
1. Dress comfortably in layered clothing.
2. Honor your modesty level.
3. Take advantage of an environment without pretenses.
4. Participate in the opportunity for healing past traumas and assuring your safety and appropriateness.

Chapter 9:

On the Massage Table at Last (Indulging All the Senses)

The therapist has taken your health history and asked what your goal is for the massage. Now she will inquire about your clothing options, choice of oils or lotions, and perhaps your music preference; she will discuss your temperature needs for the massage room, your position (lying face up or down) to start, and instruct you to lie between the two sheets. Then she will leave the room to wash her hands while you get on the table and cover yourself; and when she returns, she will ask if you are comfortable before she begins the massage.

Face Cradle

Let us start with the extension at the end of the table—this is the face cradle and it has efficient capabilities, which I talk about in upcoming paragraphs. The cutout in the cradle allows you to lie face down and breathe easily, so you do not have to torque your head to one side during your massage. Most people want to purchase face cradles for their beds after they have tried the cushioned cutouts during their massages. Unfortunately, manufacturers do not make face cradles for beds.

A face cradle can be adjusted for wider and thinner faces; as well, its angle can be positioned according to each person's need. When set appropriately, the cradle helps the receiver's neck to settle into a natural stretch—in turn, this lengthens the entire spine, creating space between the vertebrae, much like what happens to your body after a night of sleep. We are literally taller at the start of the day than at the end, because gravity compacts our spine in response to our standing for lengths of time. When small changes are made to the body in one short hour, they feel like big changes.

At the beginning of your massage and before your mind settles, you may find yourself looking through the cutout of the face cradle and being entertained by the therapist's feet, the patterns in the carpet or floor, or the curious face of a pet (if the massage is being given in a recipient's home). Eventually though, you will probably succumb to the long, slow, and deep massage strokes that soothe, relax, and coax you into closing your eyes and surrendering your head to the gentle face cradle. In later stages of your session, you may find these strokes to be convenient for snoring and even drooling; massage is one of those rare environments in which snoring and sleeping are perceived as compliments to the therapist's expertise. In fact, a recipient's sleeping during massage is seen as the ultimate act of trust in the practitioner.

Bolsters

When your body's muscles are unsupported during a massage, they must work to stay clear of the table, and this causes them unnecessary tension and strain. Providing support with bolsters and pillows accelerates relaxation in your muscles.

Here, I explain how bolsters help in a massage setting, and the reason why you might want to make more use of them when you recline and sleep. As you lie facing down, the bolster is used to fill the gap between your ankles and the table as a means of support; it also takes pressure off your ankles and clears space for your toes so they are not pressed against the table, which may cause foot cramps and discomfort.

If your legs turn out naturally, they cause your feet to roll to the side when you are face down—so the supportive bolster will take some of the twist out of your legs, but it can also prevent tension in your lower back.

When you lie facing up, a bolster placed behind the knees raises and supports them, and it helps bring the lower back in contact with the table, as a means of support. This method alone is of great comfort to you as you lie on your back. Propping your body with supportive bolsters brings immediate help for tense muscles—and the massage has not even done its part yet!

So, if you must experience the support of bolsters before your first massage even begins, or if you choose to make a lifestyle change by using bolsters, here is a tip for making your own: Take an old pillow, one that's ready to be thrown away; fold it in half lengthwise then sew the two sides together. A longer pillow is better, because if the pillow is short, you will need two bolsters, one for each leg.

Support Pillows

Now that you are on a roll with lifestyle changes acquired while receiving your massage, there are other areas of your body wishing for support—the neck, when facing up, is one of them; but as the gap behind the neck differs from person to person, choose the right fit from a variety of pillow sizes. Millet pillows are a popular treat, as they are on the larger, firmer side and good for necks desiring these qualities; and you can find these millet pillows online, in catalogs, and in stores. For necks with small gaps, however, use the can't-get-rid-of-oldie-but-goodie pillow; or use a down pillow, which is soft, sweet, and light. The last option is the creative one, easily customized for any neck, and that is a rolled up towel. Use one roll for small gaps, two for larger gaps, and so on. This option is ready and waiting in your home right now; use it to maintain the curve of your neck for a twenty-minute break, but only for short periods, as a towel can be hard to sleep on.

For large-breasted women lying face down, the pectoral area just above the breasts is another area in need of support. Placing the appropriate pillow size or towel roll in the gap above the breasts will help to relieve pressure on the breasts, making this face-down position a pleasurable experience rather than an uncomfortable one.

The towel is also supportive when one shoulder or hip is raised back slightly from the table because of tension, while the other hip continues to rest on the table. Again, filling the gap with a pillow or towel supports the muscles and helps to let go of the tension.

When you lie face down, one last place that does not have a gap but which is often happier with an extra pillow is the area beneath your belly; a pillow placed here flattens the arch in your lower back, thereby relaxing your back muscles and causing other areas to do the same.

Eye Pillows (The Smallest of the Pillows)

The eye pillow, usually made of soft silk and filled with flax seed, provides a gentle pressure for your closed eyes; and its weight, which is similar to a miniature sandbag, helps to still your restless or tired eyes from the day's events. The eye pillow darkens the room as if at bedtime, an association the body responds to in kind; however, not everyone will desire this invitation into darkness and may prefer to take the eye pillow off now and then to catch the day's light or keep things on the lighter side.

Body Support Systems

It is amazing how a body support system can feel so good although it looks so strange. This is a full body cushion that has cutouts in all the necessary places to keep your body comfortable and in correct alignment when you lie face down, face up, and on your side; and just like the pillow- and bolster-propping method, this cushion rests on top of the massage table so you can relax on it. Why then, you might ask, do we need to use the propping method when the body support cushion can do it all? The answer is simply a preference of the massage therapist, although therapists who perform pregnancy massage use these cushions so that expectant mothers can lie comfortably on their bellies and sides.

Receiving such attentiveness through these tools of support helps to nurture and customize your special time.

Selecting Music

Appropriate music is conducive to the massage setting, as it can enhance the massage and assist your receptivity; but music works for people differently, and one client taught me this truth in a way I have never forgotten. I had selected the slowest, gentlest music I owned, and thought it was the best choice for her Type A personality; however, she continued to fidget long into the massage. I tried waiting it out, assuming this day was more difficult for her to relax than other days, until she finally let out an energetic moan and complained, "Do you have anything besides that funeral music? I find it so depressing!"

So much for guessing what is best for others, regardless of my good intentions. Can you see why your feedback—whether solicited or not—is important to your receiving what you want? Unlike my expressive client, some people do find it difficult to express their preferences for fear of being labeled "fussy" or "high maintenance." This is your special time to have things your way, so it is appropriate to ask for a particular type of music, be it melodic, synthesized strings, soft piano, Native American flute, Gregorian chants, classical, or new age—common styles of music played during massage. Furthermore, you might want to bring a favorite piece of music from home, so that when you return to your own space and listen to the music again, your body will respond through association, just as it did when you heard the music during your massage. The volume at which you prefer to listen to music matters, too; and, yes, you can certainly ask that the volume be set to your liking for your massage.

But just as music has the ability to enhance a massage, it can also detract from and disrupt the gentle massage environment. For instance, if your work involves music, listening to it while receiving your massage may not be the break from routine that you need. Music should not be the primary focus of the massage; it should be an enhancer, with *you* being the focal point.

On the other hand, some massage recipients prefer no music at all. One client revealed that she likes to listen to the sounds of oil and friction made by the strokes on her skin.

Silence Is Golden

Talking is essential to human nature and it can also be habitual; sometimes we talk to fill a void or simply because it is what we do and are expected to do; indeed, it is also tempting to chat. That said, however, the massage environment is one of those few places where talking is not expected, and many clients find this a relief.

When I had a bout of laryngitis, my clients had an unexpected opportunity to experience periods of non-interaction during their massage. Although my energy was back, my voice was not, and I greeted my clients with a note, letting them know that I had laryngitis and would not be talking, but that I felt well enough to work. They were in agreement with my silence and stayed for their massages, except for one client who often talks throughout her massage—she found it difficult carrying the entire conversation and surrendered to the outcome of my silence, remaining quiet for the rest of the hour. When the massage was over, she told me that her massage was one of the best experiences she ever had, because she stopped thinking of anything after a while. Looking ahead, she wanted to be quiet for future massages, and she asked me to remind her if she forgot and started chatting.

Letting go of the day-to-day world of thought and interaction—to reside in a place of low stimulation and deep relaxation—allows one to go deeper within and contemplate; but not everyone chooses introspection and silence, and this is okay, too.

Lotions, Oils, and Aromas

Lotions and oils are helpful and pleasurable additions when used directly by the therapist for massaging the skin, and they vary in consistency, according to the technique and type of massage. Lotions are thicker than oils and work best for slower, deeper techniques, and they are suitable for clients who prefer less greasiness. Not all types of massage require oil and lotion, and if you prefer none, be sure to say so. Scented and unscented lotions and oils are also options for you; however, if you are allergic to nuts or fruit, let your therapist know, as many oils—though of high quality—are made with grape seed, apricot, almond, sesame, and other fruit and nut ingredients.

Aromatherapy: Medicinal Pleasure

A regular client of mine initially discovered me by following her nose, literally; she caught the scent of an earlier client by tracking the aroma up the elevator and into my office on the second floor. While we both worked in the same building, we had not met until our aromatic encounter that day.

When choosing an aroma for your massage, you may follow your nose or adopt a therapeutic purpose; either choice ends in medicinal pleasure. When pursuing the first route, smell a variety of scents and chose what you most resonate with or desire. Too often clients settle for "that's nice" or "okay." Some clients think they should choose something different for a change or try a different aroma each time. When my clients choose by scent, I watch their faces, and their responses to each aroma become visible, ranging from dislike to indifference, and even ecstasy. So take the opportunity to customize your special time, as my client, Carl, does with responses like "I want the one that goes with ham. Yes, clove—it has good memories *and* smells good."

The *Essential Oils Desk Reference* emphasizes this fact well: "The fragrance of an essential oil can directly affect everything from your emotional state to your lifespan." (Essential Science Publishing 2009, 8–12; hereafter cited as *Desk Reference*). When a fragrance is inhaled, it travels by way of the cilia (fine hairs lining the nostrils) and enters the limbic system of the brain. The *Desk Reference* adds: "Because the limbic system is directly connected to those parts of the brain that control heart rate, blood pressure, breathing, memory, stress levels, and hormone balance, essential oils can have profound physiological and psychological effects."

Aromatherapy not only works by smell alone but by absorption through the skin. According to the *Desk Reference,* this is because "essential oils have a unique ability to penetrate cell membranes and diffuse throughout the blood and tissues. The unique, lipid-soluble structure of essential oils is very similar to the makeup of our cell membranes. The molecules of essential oils are also relatively small, which enhances their ability to penetrate into the cells. When topically applied to the feet or elsewhere, essential oils can travel throughout the body in a matter of minutes. The ability of some essential oils, like clove, to decrease the viscosity or thickness of the blood can enhance circulation and immune function." Each aroma has a specific function, whether that is to calm the nervous system, relax the muscles, balance the emotions, and much more. Take, for instance, lavender oil and its function as explained by the *Desk Reference*: "Lavender oil has been used for burns, insect bites, headaches, PMS, insomnia, stress, and hair growth." It is easy to see why essential oils for aromatherapy enhance the benefits of massage.

Not all therapists use aromas, as some people are allergic to scents. Ask your therapist if you can bring your own scent to put on a cotton pad for your special time; and if you condition yourself to the same scent each time, you can use *that* scent at home so your body can continue to relax.

Massage offers an opportunity to explore and experience your rich inner world through all your senses. The nature of this experience is unique to each individual, however, and for this reason, no two massages are the same for anyone, not even for the client who sees the same massage therapist. A client and therapist can adopt a particular plan, but the complex *bodymind* is always gathering and assimilating information which determines the outcome and experience of a given day's massage.

Points worth rubbing in:
1. Ask for what you want regarding your massage. Go ahead and risk being "high maintenance," as this is your special time.
2. Give peace and quiet a chance.
3. Make comfort and pleasure—learned from your massages—a part of your every day, because the materials you need are all around you.

Chapter 10:
Receiving the Massage
(Feedback Is a Two-Way Process)

*T*o get a good massage you need to give good feedback, an exchange that makes every session a two-way process. This chapter explains how to give feedback and why feedback is essential in helping you receive what you need and want in a massage.

Guidelines for Determining Pressure

Your feedback is helpful to the therapist who must determine the right amount of pressure for working with your muscles—and how much pressure is right? Let me begin by saying that if your therapist works too deeply, too quickly, you could be sore the next day unnecessarily. Too much pressure may be uncomfortable for you, and the discomfort will cause your muscles to tense up; and since causing tension is counterproductive to the relaxation of your muscles, the slogan *no pain, no gain* is truly ineffective here. Tight, contracted muscles respond to pressure with resistance; they need time and the right amount of pressure to release the tension, which they hold. Your therapist will work with your pain tolerance to find the right amount of pressure, and then increase the pressure incrementally as you are able to tolerate it. On the other hand, too little pressure will not give your muscles the resistance they require to release their tension. Consequently, the muscles remain tense and contracted.

The following guidelines can help you communicate your desired pressure levels:

1. When the pressure is just right, you will know because it *hurts so good*. This feeling is often expressed with a long sigh, accompanied by the release of tense muscles; this sigh is familiar verbiage to a massage therapist, and no other explanation is necessary by you.

2. How do you arrive at a *hurt so good* feeling? Many therapists use a standard one-to-ten scale to determine your pleasure and pain perceptions, with ten being the most pain and, one, the least; seven would be the optimum pressure.

There are different schools of thought on the topic of pressure and pain; some therapists and clients believe that pain is necessary to get results, while others do not. More crucial to your success than the issue of pain, however, is the type of massage you are receiving and the reason for the massage, and both points are to be taken into consideration. A relaxing massage for some people means a light touch; whereas, for others, deep pressure is required to get to a state of relaxation. You may need to experiment in order to determine the right pressure for a specific outcome, and then find the therapist whose technique supports your belief system. It is possible for you to want deep pressure on one occasion and a light touch during the next; so it is important to know what you need, and make sure to express that to your therapist.

Your Therapist's Feedback

In addition to inquiring about pressure levels, your therapist may give you feedback about what she observes. For instance, when you are lying face down, she may observe that one of your hips rests on the table while the other does not, which may indicate that your pelvis is rotated. Although this may sound alarming, it is quite common. Rotation can happen when muscles in the buttocks or lower back are tighter on one side, causing the pelvis to torque or rotate; however, massage can help release the tension, and restore the correct posture. If tight muscles do not cause this rotation, the culprit could be skeletal-related; the vertebrae in that area of the spine could be misaligned, which is also common. In this case, your therapist may suggest that you see your chiropractor to realign your pelvis, or she may recommend a chiropractor if you do not have one. Receiving a chiropractic adjustment as soon as possible after your massage is highly recommended, because the skeleton moves with greater ease and holds the adjustment better when it is freed up from tight muscles.

The practitioner will also use your breath to gather information from your body. In general, when an area is tight, there is a tendency to hold your breath and avoid breathing into that area of tension. Your therapist may have you inhale and focus your breath on the area in which she is applying pressure; the act of inhaling and exhaling causes the muscle to expand and contract, which in turn, releases the holding pattern.

A healthy muscle does two things: it works, and it rests. When a muscle is at rest, it expands, allowing blood to flow easily and supply the oxygen and nutrients that are necessary for its proper functioning. When a muscle works, it contracts, and this contraction serves as a pump for expelling lactic acid and toxins, flushing them from the system; contraction also helps return the blood to the heart, which is a significant benefit of massage.

However, muscles do not always function optimally, and they remain tight or contracted chronically even when our bodies are at rest or during sleep. Tight muscles restrict the flow of blood and limit necessary nutrients and oxygen. Chronically tense muscles become fatigued as a result of working overtime, causing other muscles to work in their place; if the problem is not resolved, a domino effect occurs, until a muscle group fatigues and there is overall weakness. In this syndrome, a person wakes up tired after a night of sleep because the muscles never rested fully; and this is also the person who says, "I'm falling apart! First my back was tight and sore, then my shoulders and neck, and now it's my arms and legs." Such a statement describes the basic fact that the body is an integrated system. I tell my clients that we first learned this fact in the words of a children's song, "Dry Bones," in which we connect the ankle bone to the leg bone, the leg bone to the knee bone, the knee bone to the thigh bone, and the thigh bone to the hip bone, and so on. Indeed, the body *is* an integrated system.

Stating Your Needs

No matter how many resources you have to give feedback or no matter how much experience you have with receiving massage, you may find that once you lie down and relax during the massage, initiating a conversation seems too much; consequently, this is why you'll want to state your needs before the massage begins. Your therapist will check in with you from time to time, asking questions like "Is this what you are wanting?" or "How is this pressure?" At which point you need only respond with monosyllabic answers such as *yes*, *no*, *more*, *less*, *ah*, and so on.

While receiving your massage, you may realize how tired you are, and the quiet, safe environment may lull you to sleep; if falling asleep is what you need or want, then do so. Sometimes, even if you are not tired, you may respond to the massage by resting deeply. This is your body's way of receiving the information, and it is best that you and your therapist honor your body's response. Should this happen to you, sharing feedback after your massage is more appropriate.

The Body-Mind Process

Because deep relaxation often occurs during massage, it is common for a recipient to enter the alpha state, a state of physical and mental relaxation while you are awake and aware of what is happening around you. In this state, memory recall and problem solving come more easily, and, therefore, the alpha state may be used intentionally during massage for a specific purpose. The following exchange is a good example of the body-mind connection and how both affect each other; as well, it shows the role that massage can play if you choose to use massage in this way:

Amy's body-mind session. Partway into her massage, Amy recalled a dream she had the previous night and shared it as though the dream were taking place in the moment:

And there on my kitchen floor I see him, fear, and hate him, try not to look at him. I cannot keep myself from looking at him. With each sideways peek at him, his eyes pierce through me, follow me wherever I go.

Just a short distance from me is his small, round, bloated, and pasty-skinned bald head with icy-blue eyes. He sits on a base, clattering around my linoleum floor like a set of dentures let loose. He is grotesque in every way....

Amy: Now on the massage table I remember my dream. I flashback on the grotesque head. Yes, my dream last night, I had forgotten.

Therapist: [*While massaging*] Do you want to explore it?

Amy: Yes.

Therapist: How can he consume your attention and yet be the head of a body only...and small as well? [*She brings Amy's attention to her breath. Amy thinks about this and pauses awhile.*]

Therapist: Notice your breath right now. What is it doing?

Amy: I notice I'm barely breathing, more like I'm holding my breath.

Therapist: Do you know why you're breathing this way?

Amy: All I know is I'm afraid of him, he scares me.

Therapist: Do you notice this response to fear by holding your breath, and how your muscles tighten to hold your breath?

Amy: Yes, that's where I've been achy.

Therapist: Take some slow, deep breaths and push my hands up with your breath. Go only as far as it feels comfortable.

Amy: I do. After doing this awhile, my body feels better and less achy. I realize I wasn't aware of my body but only of the tension until now.

Therapist: In this relaxed state, knowing you are safe, let's revisit the head. How do you feel now?

Amy: I laughed when I recalled him, and I laughed at myself. When I recalled how I felt earlier I realized it was my undivided attention that gave him such power, my power. Power to judge me, which consumed me totally. He *was* me!

Therapist: Why did he judge you?

Amy: Upon reflection, I had been hard on myself around the time of the dream. I had been heartless in fact, to the extent that things got out of proportion. I was so consumed with self criticism and judgment for the way I was handling some things.

Therapist: Does this happen often?

Amy: Unfortunately, yes, other people tell me that too, that I'm being hard on myself before I realize it.

Therapist: Then these achy back muscles between your shoulders and around your heart are your barometer, your friendly reminder that the judge is back. [*She emphasizes them by deepening Amy's pressure.*] You can do what you learned today; breathe deeply, have self-compassion, and feel more comfortable in your body.

Amy: That sounds good to me.

Nancy's body-mind session. Here is another example of an interactive body-mind session, recounted in client Nancy's own words:

> I did not personally believe in the body-mind connection until I experienced it unexpectedly one afternoon with Debra.
>
> As Debra massaged my legs, we began talking about my high school girlfriend and her family, a loud and large Italian family. I described how my friend's four brothers and their noisy gatherings were alien to me, since I grew up in a quiet family of four girls. Debra commented on the tenseness in my legs that occurred when I spoke of these boys; I felt I was fighting

against Debra's touch and I could not relax my legs. Debra inquired about my relationship with my friend's brother, and I admitted I had felt a certain degree of sexual tension with them—one in particular. Debra maintained soft contact with my legs while asking me if I experienced these feelings of sexual tension with anyone else, and I admitted that two men in particular affected me in the same way.

I had repressed sexuality hidden away in my legs, especially in my thighs; and although I was able to draw the connection between my memories and my body, I still could not let go of the tension and relax. Debra told me that my awareness was the first and biggest step for addressing these kinds of issues. I felt safe and secure with her, and I also felt comfortable to simply *be* with my tension at that moment. Before this occurrence, I never realized the extent of difficult memories held in my body that could be brought alive again and understood through touch.

Points worth rubbing in:

1. To get a good massage, give good feedback.
2. Breath is golden.
3. State your needs beforehand.
4. Be open to your therapist's feedback.
5. Breath and awareness deepen a connection to yourself and your massage.
6. Massage can be a time for introspection, insight, and integration, whether verbally or non-verbally.
7. Your body is like a barometer; there is much information in your tension and pain.

The Feared and Unexpected

Gas. We all have flatulence, yes, but what an inopportune time to encounter it, when here you are receiving your massage and most likely contracting your muscles to retain the gas from expelling. Tensing and worrying led to your massage in the first place. So why withhold them now? And what do you do about your gas? You release it, let it go, that's what. Some clients choose to announce it to the therapist before releasing it, while others do not, and the therapist ignores the act and simply moves on; if necessary, the therapist may leave the room momentarily. Once again, remember that the massage environment is unlike the usual social setting.

Erections. While the notion of becoming aroused during massage is a common concern for men, erections happen rarely, as a matter of fact. This is because massage helps to override arousal with its relaxing qualities and with the therapist's professional attitude and use of words, which keep the client's mind focused on the healing and on any therapeutic goals.

Massage therapists often begin their massages with relaxing techniques and by having clients lie face down, because nervousness and anxiety can exasperate recipients and provoke unwanted responses from them. As nervousness subsides and as relaxation prevails to become the primary response, earlier fears and concerns diminish too.

It is true that thoughts and fantasies affect sexual arousal and stimulation, and if this is the cause of your arousal, then focusing your thoughts elsewhere will create a change. Here is one man's experience along these lines:

This is Paul's Story.

There is no escaping the fact that massage and erotic thoughts are easily linked in the minds of most men. Lying naked under a sheet, bathed in soft light, relaxing to gentle music while another person massages your well-oiled body, is enough to put most men's minds into the land of sexual fantasy. I think it is probably a very normal mental reaction for the person who is experiencing massage for the first few times. It certainly was with me. In fact, erections and the inner panic and embarrassment they caused were part of my early massages, and these diminished the experience and benefits of each session considerably.

At the time, I was very concerned with these thoughts. They caused me a great deal of mental discomfort and embarrassment. Did my therapist think I was a pervert? Did this happen to other people? Maybe massage wasn't for me?

Fortunately, I was seeing an excellent and experienced massage therapist who was untroubled by what she saw as a very human reaction to a new experience. Before we began, she would relax me with conversation before I got on the table. By beginning the massage in a comfortable and professional setting, I was able to begin to grasp what the massage experience could be <u>if I let it.</u> And although she and I never spoke of my fantasies, I did speak with some close friends about it and they assured me that the thoughts I was having were perfectly normal and not at all unique. Learning this from people I trusted was a relief to me.

Still, I was uncomfortable whenever sexual thoughts or fantasies invaded my thinking while I was on the table. But I was also aware that during each massage I was beginning to grasp a better understanding of the wonderful freeing experience that massage therapy could bring. As I began to allow myself to enjoy the nuances that each new massage brought, the sexual imagery began to fade. In time, I came to very much resent the erotic fantasies that interrupted my tranquility and serenity on the table, and so I began to exercise my mind and was able to push the disruptive thoughts aside and enjoy the deep physical, emotional, and spiritual benefits that massage offers. As I lay on the table deep in thought and perhaps for the first time in my life enjoying a true meditative experience, I began to under-stand the ability that massage has to mend and restore the balance in a person's life.

Now, my massage sessions are far too important to me to have them disrupted by jangling physical fantasies that in no way reflect the reality of the situation. Sexual thoughts still arrive unannounced during my massage, but they are fleeting and easily dismissed.

Points worth rubbing in:

1. Erections and arousal are a natural response to plea-sure. Relaxation overrides stimulating responses.
2. Deep, slow breathing is one of life's greatest tools for letting go of physical tension and mental anxiety. Indulge abundantly.
3. Use your mind to focus on relaxing qualities.

Emotions

The massage environment can provide emotional safety and support. Sometimes emotions catch us by surprise and sometimes they have difficulty finding release. This is because emotions undergo a ripening process, and release only when they are ready; part of their readiness and timing involves the right situation and the right cause. Be assured that emotions are appropriate to the massage setting, if you so choose to express them.

Many of us share the tendency to resist or deny our full range of emotions, and we may find diversions from our emotional pain through excessive eating, shopping, exercising, sex, and working, to name a few. We may even project these emotions onto people we care about, causing them hurt just as we also hurt ourselves. If we succeed in denying and resisting our emotions, our feelings become vague or frozen, making these emotions more difficult to identify, access, and release. Such frozen feelings affect our ability to feel emotions in general, even positive emotions like joy and love. Joe Weldon, a Master Rubenfeld Synergist, states it this way, *"The range of motion in a body is equal to the range of emotion. This means that if there is great joy in a body then there will be great movement of that body. If there is great sadness in a body, there will be very little or no movement of that body. The body instead will be weighted and stuck. When we touch and open up the range of motion in a body, we allow space for the experience and expression of the emotions"* (J. Weldon, *pers. comm.*, June 2011).

Emotional pain is similar to physical pain. For instance, if a rib is out of alignment, you may have pain when breathing, using your arms, and resting them at your sides; your pain remains until the bone is put back where it belongs. The pain is heightened when it is being adjusted, but then relief follows. The only pain remaining is the soreness where the rib was out of alignment; and the longer the rib has been out of alignment, the more sore and raw that area will be. However, in time, all the soreness heals.

Emotions respond similarly. During the period when they are not addressed, emotions may cause pain or even inhibit joy, and you may hear yourself—or someone else—uttering responses such as the following: "That's just the way I am," or "I never used to be this way, but now I am a resentful person," or "I'm not one to cry," and "I only cry at movies."

Emotional baggage responds like a congested or blocked system; it may affect relationships, enjoyable work, and quality time off—and suppressed emotions worsen without an outlet. For example, recall an instance when you suppressed laughter at a time when it was inappropriate to express it. Did the feelings inside you build or subside?

When facilitating the release of emotions as a massage therapist, I have learned the difference between causing someone pain in contrast to accessing and releasing the pain already held within that person. My assistance is similar to the chiropractor's effort in helping put a misaligned rib back in its proper place. Some people find it easier to access and release emotions through body-centered therapy such as massage, while others find that the combination of both psychotherapy and massage work better together than either practice on its own.

Releasing withheld emotions in a safe, supportive environment can be a profound and even life-changing experience. Those who have experienced this liberation report that resisting the emotions was more painful than releasing them. You can heal the emotions you allow yourself to feel, no matter the extent of these emotions.

Points worth rubbing in:

1. Unreleased emotions can manifest in physical symptoms and inhibit other emotions.
2. It is more painful to withhold and suppress emotions than it is to experience, release, and express them productively and in a safe environment.
3. The intensity of a particular emotional issue lessens with each release.
4. Emotions are part of being human.

Visuals

Not everyone responds to massage in the same way, but many do see colors and images. While working in a day spa, I treated a client of mine, Katie, who was scheduled for a three-hour appointment with me; her session included a massage, salt glow, eucalyptus steam bath, seaweed scalp treatment, and a paraffin back de-stressing treatment. This was her first experience with these therapies.

During Katie's seaweed scalp treatment, I massaged her head, and while the seaweed was setting, I moved down to her feet and began doing an energy system called Reiki (see Chapter 4). There is no movement with Reiki, only the light laying of hands. Katie sat up suddenly to look for me, although I was kneeling at her feet with my palms on them.

"I'm right here," I assured her. "Did you think I left the room?"

"No, I knew you were here," Katie answered back. "I thought I fell asleep, but I've been awake. It's just that I suddenly feel so alert, still relaxed but mentally clear. I never felt this way before."

We shampooed the seaweed out of her hair, and then applied the hot paraffin on her back. While the wax set, I continued with the Reiki. Katie told me she was seeing many images and proceeded to describe them to me. The first was an image of black and white clouds in the sky, but the sun became increasingly intense until it burned the clouds away completely. In place of the clouds, a still image of her family appeared, and everyone was together including her extended family. Then other family members she did not know joined in. She said they seemed like the family of the world.

Katie's second image was of beautiful and unusual fruit; they were odd and large-shaped, blue and purple with white tops. She had never seen anything like them before, and thought they must be from a different planet.

The last image she saw was a face that was made up of hundreds of rivers, and each river was very thin with different shades of blue. A sunset cast its hue over some areas.

Katie told me she had no idea something as profound as this could happen, and she would need time to assimilate it before coming back for more. As a painter, she intended to go home and paint the images that had come to her. Although seeing images of varying degrees is common during a massage, the complexity of Katie's images is uncommon. Perhaps, it is so because she is an artist.

Some people find it difficult to retain the image while verbalizing it. In this case, it is helpful to follow the visual in silence rather than risk losing it altogether. Some choose to share it afterwards, and others keep the visuals to themselves. Still others find that speaking about the image while seeing it enhances their process, and this helps them stay conscious of its unfolding.

The world of massage has many rich surprises (for giver and receiver), especially when suspending judgment and expectation. Images may be complex or they may be as simple as a small purple light. This light may inspire an insight, emotion, or sensation; or it may simply be entertaining. As one of my clients put it: "I'm just lying here enjoying the light show with my eyes closed."

Chapter 11:
Post-Massage Care
(Invest in Your Investment)

How you treat yourself after the massage is just as important as the massage itself. Invest in your investment, be gentle and nurturing with yourself, and drink plenty of water. When muscles relax, toxins release from tight muscles and tissue in your system, and flushing them with plenty of water is recommended. An Epsom salt bath also draws out toxins and soothes sore tissue. Soreness is more likely for those who do not get regular massages or have not been exercising regularly. Neutral, tempered water is the most relaxing, whereas hot water can be fatiguing when used to an extreme. Any soreness from the massage should subside within 24 to 48 hours, and if it persists beyond that, contact your therapist for guidance.

You may feel emotionally sensitive or vulnerable after a massage, without your usual tight muscles as armor. Place yourself in a favorable environment afterwards, so you can process anything that may have surfaced during the session; this is beneficial, as is writing your experience in a journal or capturing it through another art form.

A gentle, easy walk helps the body, mind, and emotions integrate the work done during the massage. Strenuous physical activities could undo any benefits from your session; therefore, it is wise not to schedule your massage close to regular workouts, activities, and responsibilities. Some clients even take the next morning or day off from work, a decision that many may perceive as extravagant or overindulgent, although others prefer to call it self care. The more you nurture yourself the healthier and happier you are.

With so much transformation taking place within a session, you may not be sure what you are feeling. If you believe something adverse resulted from the massage, call your massage therapist and ask; too often, clients do not call back, and pertinent information is lost to the massage therapist who has no other way of knowing and could use the information for future sessions. The client endures unnecessary pain or concern, and a client-therapist relationship may be broken if the client chooses not to return because of this.

Furthermore, the benefits from your massage do not need to stop when the massage does; cultivate these benefits instead. Perhaps, your therapist suggested exercises, visualizations, affirmations, reading material, and ergonomic or lifestyle changes. Perhaps, you captured an insight of your own, so set it in motion while clarity and motivation are strong. Make what you learn from your massages a lifestyle.

Now that you have experienced transformation through massage, do not stop; keep going, as things have been set in motion. Sometimes a follow up session within a couple of days is appropriate to see a change through. Your body did not arrive in its current state in a session's timeframe; likewise, it does not transform within that session. Ironically, when the body is in the process of healing, it may feel worse before it feels better. I illustrate my point in the following example: If you wear your shoes on the wrong feet by mistake, your feet feel uncomfortable even after you correct the error, but the tissues of your feet continue to resist the correction just as they begin to adapt to a healthier direction. Emotional changes behave like this, too. Perhaps, an emotional issue surfaced during your session; an interruption can upset you and cause you confusion and pain. My point being that you would not want to stop any support for your body-mind process, just as you would not stop taking a prescription drug before its prescribed dosage period ends. The timing for processing physical and emotional issues varies among people; some issues and clients need more time than others do. Discuss the timing for future sessions with your therapist, including discussions of the best types of massage or alternative health care for situations as they arise. Life continues to offer its challenges, so why not support it with ongoing assistance through the numerous types of alternative care available to you.

Points worth rubbing in:
1. Invest in your investment; practice post-massage self care.
2. Schedule massage appointments wisely around physical workouts and your other responsibilities.

Chapter 12:

Wrapping It Up
(Scheduling Your Next Massage, Tipping, and Cancellations)

Scheduling Your Next Massage

While basking in the benefits of your massage, being aware of its full value, and undiminished by all that awaits you on the other side of the door, go ahead and schedule your next session.

Your sincere intentions to schedule at a later date may be delayed long past the time you would have received your next session, unless you scheduled ahead, of course. Life has a way of getting by us, however, because when you call your therapist to set up an appointment, there may be a further delay if her schedule is busy or if your appointment time is a popular one.

How often should you receive a massage? If money and time are not an issue, weekly massages are excellent maintenance for body, mind, and emotions; otherwise, let your body guide you. If your concern is physical, keep ahead of pains and restrictions that were relieved from previous massage sessions. To break a chronic cycle, receive your next massage *before* you feel the same pains returning; obviously, this process may involve trial and error, and the same stands true for the relief of mental and emotional patterns. Massage is very useful for breaking habitual patterns, whether they are physical, mental, or emotional.

The psyche likes knowing when good things are coming—like weekends, vacations, special occasions, and, yes, massage too. Knowing when the next session will be, soothes the nervous system and provides a coping method for life's challenges in the meantime. Furthermore, instead of calling to schedule your next appointment, you can ask your therapist to call you around a particular date when you would like to schedule a session.

When scheduling, remember to choose a time that will keep you from doing anything taxing afterwards; physical workouts following a massage could undo the relaxation benefits you have received and may result in your poor workout performance. Allow at least a couple of hours before heading for your workout, if you must do so on the same day of your massage. Likewise, to earn the full benefits of massage, attend to your errands long before your session or a few hours following it, or do your errands at a different time. In other words, *invest in your investment*.

Tipping

There is no simple answer regarding tipping in the field of massage. Unlike services at restaurants and beauty salons that follow a general percentage range for tipping, massage tips vary greatly according to the type of massage, the location in which it is received, and the massage therapist involved in the transaction.

The reason for this undefined reward amount is that massage falls into two categories: medical and service. Just as chiropractors and other health practitioners do not receive tips, massage therapists working in this setting do not expect tips either.

However, medically-related massages are not the only types of services performed in these offices. Some massages may begin that way, when a client has a prescription for massage therapy from a physician. After the prescription is completed, the client often chooses to continue receiving massages at the same location (having built a rapport with a massage therapist) and decides to stay on for stress reduction and relaxation massage. This transitional type of massage falls into the service category related to tipping, and shows how easily massage and tipping can become complicated; it is the reason why clients remain confused about tipping or, perhaps, have never considered it.

Another situation that factors in is whether the therapist is a proprietor, employee, or independent contractor. Therapists employed at spas, beauty salons, hotels, retreats, and chiropractors' offices receive a percentage of the massage fee being charged, and this percentage varies, depending on the environment and arrangement the therapist has made with the employer. In general, a massage therapist's cut is 50%–60% of the original massage fee, so in this case the practitioner may rely on tips to bolster the low wages. What, you may ask is a healthy tip? To this, I would say, a fifteen percent tip of the massage fee is a good place to start. Independent contractors also receive a percentage cut that varies, and they must deduct their own taxes, although they may or may not depend on tips to support their income. Therapists working for themselves set their fee according to what they need; therefore, they do not expect tips to make up for their income, and may or may not accept tips when offered. This is a personal preference and varies among therapists.

It is common for the same massage therapist to work in more than one environment within the same day or week. For instance, I had a private practice on the second floor of a three-story professional building, but also did massage therapy three mornings each week for a chiropractor on the first floor; for five days a week, I saw private massage clients in my own office. I was a proprietor and an employee in the same day, doing the same work in both locations—one setting was a medical environment, while the other was a private office space.

As you can see, there are no clear guidelines for tipping with massage, and it is best to assess the situation with this information in mind; offer your therapist a tip if you so desire, and then wait for a response.

Cancellations

Life gets busy and cancellations do happen. Too often, coveted times that we reserve for ourselves are forfeited to other responsibilities, or the times are exchanged for other pleasurable offers. If compromises cannot be made and cancellations are necessary, schedule your next session at the time that you cancel.

In addition, by your giving as much notice in advance as possible, you become mindful of your massage therapist and others waiting for an appointment. Twenty-four hours is a standard block of time to make a cancellation, but more notice helps all parties to reconnect, as it takes time for people involved to receive and return messages. Often, twenty-four hours is *not* enough time to make up for an unexpected cancellation.

Some therapists ask for a full or partial fee with less than twenty-four hours notice, because the time reserved for you is lost income for the practitioner without this fee. Unlike salary positions, therapists are paid only when they perform their work and not because they showed up. Additionally, because of an unexpected cancellation, another client who might want the time slot allocated for you will not be able to receive a massage, so being considerate keeps a relaxed and respectful relationship with your therapist.

If you must cancel, a win-win option is to gift your session to someone else, and everyone receives something this way. You feel better for your gesture, the recipient is happy to have a massage, and your therapist is compensated for the time you reserved in advance.

Points worth rubbing in:

1. Schedule your next massage before departing at the end of your current session.
2. Assess the situation for tipping, and ask if you are unsure.
3. When you need to cancel your appointment, give plenty of notice, so those waiting for an appointment have time to take your place, and your therapist's time and income can also be compensated.

All-inclusive Checklist of Considerations

1. When preparing to establish a relationship with a massage therapist, do consider the practitioner's location, her days and hours of operation, and the types of massage being offered that can meet your needs.
2. When making appointments, communicate any conditions that the therapist should be cautious of, and reiterate these conditions upon your arrival and before receiving your massage.

3. Ask your insurance company about coverage for massage; as well, if there are discounts through a medical extension plan. Bring insurance forms to your massage appointment if a therapist's signature is required.

4. Ask the massage establishment or massage therapist about fees, sliding scales, and any discounts.

5. Allow plenty of time to get to your appointment, and go unhurried.

6. Eat lightly before your massage.

7. Remember to bring your gift certificate, cash, or checkbook with you.

8. Handle communications beforehand, so you can be unavailable (in good conscience) during your massage.

9. Bring a favorite piece of calming music to listen to during your massage.

10. Plan a transition time after your massage to take full advantage of the benefits.

11. Bring extra clothing for your massage time (bathing trunks or bathing suit), and comfortable clothing to dress in afterwards if you arrive in nice business clothes; bring warm coat, hat, and gloves for cooler weather, and because you will want to remain warm and relaxed leaving the nurturing massage environment.

12. When receiving your massage, keep a two-way feedback system, asking for what you need.

13. Schedule your next massage before you leave; ask your therapist when and what type of work would be most beneficial to you following your session.

14. Give at least twenty-four hours notice if you need to cancel an appointment.

15. Take what you learn from your massage time and make it a lifestyle.

Chapter 13:
Integrating Massage with Alternative and Conventional Medicine

We have entered a time where Eastern (Alternative) and Western (Conventional) medicines are combining services for a broader and more wholesome approach to healthcare that can be mindful of the "whole being." In fact, the online 2009 AMTA Consumer Survey Fact Sheet has this to say: "Thirty-two percent of Americans get massages for medical and health reasons...compared to 31 percent last year."

Medicine's Contribution to Healthcare

Complementary and Alternative Medicine (CAM) is defined online by the National Center for Complementary and Alternative Medicine as "a group of diverse medical and health care systems, practices, and products that are not generally considered part of conventional medicine" (NCCAM 2011, under "Defining CAM"). Some of these systems and practices include: Massage, Osteopathy,

Chiropractic, Kinesiology, Acupuncture, Hypnosis, Naturopathy, Homeopathy, Herbology, Aromatherapy, Tai Chi, Qigong, and Yoga.

Whether an illness is treated with either alternative or conventional means, *diagnosis* is conventional medicine's significant contribution to the health field, and *diagnosis* is crucial for treatment. Another significant contribution of conventional medicine is surgery, and some progressive hospitals now augment the patient's bedside care with alternative medicine. How better to support a patient through his or her fears, concerns, and pre- and post-surgical recuperation than with a trained volunteer to listen deeply to that person, meditate with him or her, and massage or guide the patient through a positive scenario with this life event.

Your Contribution to the Healing Process

It is important to find a practitioner and treatment you can trust, and when you do succeed, trust the process and be willing to impart useful information about your situation to your practitioner. Ask for what you need and want, and do your part in the healing process, whether it involves diet and exercise or if you are required to observe your symptoms and feelings along the way, relaying them to your practitioner(s) when needed. Keep in mind, any regimen may involve a lifestyle change, which will take time to adapt to and maintain. Also keep in mind that Complementary and Alternative Medicine (CAM) often works more gradually than conventional medicine does, because not only is the body involved, but the emotions, mind, and spirit are involved too; furthermore, CAM treatments are more subtle than conventional medicine and, therefore, may take longer to show results. CAM's process of healing requires patience and mindfulness, and too often we focus on one particular outcome that is yet to be, only to ignore what we may have received thus far—qualities of calmness, better sleep, less pain, improved concentration and balance, more self-awareness which leads to healthier choices, a better attitude, and our ability to handle challenges.

Many of this book's guidelines can also be applied to your search for other alternative health practitioners and their fields of expertise such as those mentioned above. The resources to you are abundant. Take advantage of all there is to offer, because your well-being is important. I hope the information in this book will get you to the massage table and to the family of alternative medicine practitioners sooner than later.

Points worth rubbing in:
1. Find a practitioner and treatment you can trust, then trust the process.
2. Be trustworthy in imparting useful information to your practitioner.
3. Ask for what you need.
4. Be aware of and communicate your symptoms along the way.
5. Do your part by making necessary lifestyle changes.
6. Combine modalities when appropriate.

≈

The qualities of transformation, interconnection, and gratitude best summarize what the field of massage has taught me as a client and therapist during these past thirty years.

The sign on my office door reads "Transformation In Progress," because *that* is what happens on many levels; but change is not isolated to one part of the body or to one person. Just as the knee bone is connected to the thigh bone, and the thigh bone is connected to the hip bone, the body, mind, emotions, and spirit are connected too. Indeed, we all are connected to one another; thus, one person's healing and transformation, one person's sense of well-being, can affect others physically and energetically.

I am truly grateful for all that I have received from my clients, practitioners, students, friends and family in the continuous hoop of giving and receiving; and I marvel again and again at the fact that giving and receiving are not separate acts but, rather, parts of each other. I would like to close by returning to the massage setting with this last common scenario of gratitude: After seeing my client to the door, I return to the massage room to put fresh sheets on the massage table in preparation for the next person, and I find that my client has neatly smoothed and straightened the used sheets, and lovingly placed the eye pillow atop the neck pillow at the head of the massage table.

Chapter 14:
More Massage Stories

W hile writing this book, I asked my clients to share their massage experiences, and because they were clients of mine, you will notice that my name appears in most of the stories that follow. I hope these stories will speak to you in some way and bring you closer to experiencing massage, whether it is for the first time or for many more.

Adrian's story. This first story was written by a client of mine, Adrian, who works ten- to twelve-hour days, five days a week, and sometimes on weekends. She often verbalizes her gratitude for "massage day." I asked Adrian to write down what she gets from her massage, and this is her experience as she told it to me over a cup of tea in the waiting room right after her session—otherwise it would not have been written, Adrian insisted. She said the following:

> I get a massage for my mind, my spirit, and my body. If I don't put the three together, my body won't be able to feel it. It's more like going beyond the physical realm. It's really deep.

This is the thing that I do for myself now. I used to get psychotherapy and Reiki attunements. Massage helps me to catch up with myself, to reflect on the week. I don't know how much I've done during the week until I come to the massage. It is like a thermometer to know if I've been good or bad with myself.

It's a lot of things. It's talking, it's laughing, it's breathing, it's [the] quiet. When I'm relaxed, I don't care what I'm saying; I just say it.

Mark's story. When I asked Mark if he would write about a particular session for me, he had already captured the purity of the moment in his journal. Mark has received many massages over the past several years; he is an athlete (who keeps a daily journal), and a technical writer by profession. The following is his journal entry:

Today, I had a most remarkable massage. Debra had given me other massages. My body was responding to the treatments.

To start, there was nothing different. For forty minutes, stiffness was melted away. Stubborn, my shoulder blade was rigid and unyielding. Debra pressed deeply into the problem spot. Pain transmitted down my body. My arm throbbed. My legs tingled knowingly. The rigidity remained. This resistance was especially determined.

Again, the deep tension was pointedly pressed. It let loose. My hands and feet gushed with perspiration. My heart pounded. My body was numb. Cold air felt warm.

Remaining adjustments were automatic. My body twitched, altering itself every few seconds. Re-calibration sequenced throughout: arms, legs, lips, and toes included.

Adjustment slowed toward 20 minutes. Refreshed, yet weakened, my lip twitched unconsciously. My hands trembled.

Altered awareness: Single-mindedly, pre-sleep consciousness peers down a straight and empty highway crossing a barren desert. Purposefully, there is progression through an uncluttered landscape. Movement is satisfaction enough.

Debra laid her hands upon my chest. Eyes closed, my vision warmed to the fluorescent green glow of eddying and boiling streams. Aurora Borealis danced and swirled beneath my eyelids. I feared opening my eyes for loss of the display.

Debra removed her hands. The display withdrew. My senses peaked. I'm aware of the silences between the creaking. A new equilibrium has me grounded and at ease.

Aletha's story.

A massage to me is allowing myself a piece of reality in both the physical and mental realms. All day long, I'm involved in catering to other people's needs. Mentally, I set myself ready for everyone else's problems, concerns, and, once in a while, their excitement. Physically, my body must perform various tasks involving lifting, bending, standing, pushing, and speed. This is the reality of my job, but not *my* reality.

To lie on a table almost naked, motionless, surrounded by soothing sounds of nature and rhythmic beats of music playing, helps me to breathe.

For one hour, I am into me. My mind is at rest, my body is still, and I can now feel the blood warm through my veins. My whole self in sync, in its reality. Hands of healing melt away all knots, and stress levels decrease.

Rachielle's story.

Nothing had prepared me for the rigors of motherhood. Waking up every half hour or so around the clock to feed and care for a baby was the biggest challenge of my life. While I love my baby so much, there were times I was too tired to respond to his cry.

One day, Debra came to see the new baby. Noah locked his gaze on her, especially when he received a foot rub. As Debra left, she suggested I go to her office for a massage. It was the first time in two months that I ever left Noah, my baby, for more than half an hour. Debra played music that reminded me of the wind swishing through a bamboo grove. She kneaded my shoulder and my neck, and relief swooped over me. She touched a point behind my neck and asked me to drop my head to the pillow. I felt the pressure of a thousand headaches drift away in that instant. The rest of the massage was as soothing.

Knots of tension loosened in my lower back, where I felt the greatest pain during childbirth. The rest of my body proclaimed its thanks to Debra.

Today, massage plays an important role in my relationship. A simple back rub at the end of a long day is as intimate as a kiss. Even Noah expects his foot rub with joy. Debra's gift of touch stays with my family years after the first visit.

Susan's story.

I think that if there is a Heaven it would be an eternal massage. A massage with no ending, and no obligation to give anything back, just to receive.

I started having regular massages when I was driving 85 miles each way to a job. I knew I would need it to manage the stress in my shoulders. When the position ended I decided to continue seeing Debra every four weeks for a massage. It is my regular time to "check in" with her and reflect on how I am doing, how happy I am, how my life events—and those of my family—are affecting my body. And my time to relax. My only disappointment is that it ends. I try not to be too aware that the progress of the massage along my body means that it will end. I try to focus on visualizing the tension leaving my body through Debra's hands.

Several years ago, I closed my plant store in Portland, Oregon. The experience was awful because people were buying the last plants and the fixtures and asking for all the details of the demise even though they hadn't supported the store when it was in operation. I felt like they were picking my bones. At the end of the last day, I spend some time in my bathtub ridding myself of that violated feeling. I lie there imagining that all that contamination was flowing out of my fingertips. I visualized it flowing downhill to the river that passed through the city, into the Columbia River, on to the coast, and into the Pacific Ocean. It worked. I felt it was gone.

Tara's story.

I had always thought of a massage as pure indulgence. Many years before, I had received a massage of my face and neck during a facial I'd received, and it was heavenly. The lights were dimmed, there was a soft New Age type music playing, my esthetician talked so soft she practically whispered. I think I fell asleep. Unfortunately, life got more complicated with a stressful job, two children, a husband, and a house to care for, and a massage was a luxury I never indulged in. Finally, while making a reservation for a weekend away to celebrate our sixteenth anniversary, I decided I would celebrate with a massage for myself, while my husband golfed.

The receptionist at the Spa booked me with a male therapist, Gary. My first thought, but I never said anything, was that I would have preferred a woman. I wondered if it would sound strange to request a woman. Needless to say, I never did, and I later convinced myself that fate had a way of working and that I should just leave the appointment alone.

The morning of my appointment, I arrived early to take a steam bath as suggested. While in the locker room, women were entering, making comments to each other about how great their massages were. I was really feeling relaxed and was anticipating a wonderful experience, thinking I should have done this sooner. While waiting at the receptionist's desk, I observed the other massage therapists meeting their clients. They were all women...very soft spoken and gentle. Then Gary arrived. He had the demeanor of a tennis instructor: very lively and energetic. He escorted me to the room. A CD was playing classical music, but not a soothing piece with strings and flutes...it was heavy percussion and piano. He never asked what I'd like to listen to...and of course I never said. As my massage began, he proceeded to talk, and I learned all about his life, but I would have preferred dimmer lights and quiet. At one point I told him he was pressing too hard, and that it was hurting a bit, and he eased up for awhile. Later, just as I was about to mention again that it was hurting a bit he informed me he was giving me a deeper massage because it was more effective.

I left feeling very disappointed. I had the experience of a prize fighter going into the ring, rather than the meditative, restorative experience I was after. As I was exiting the room, a woman was leaving the room next door. She told me she felt disoriented she was so relaxed and loose... I had to point out where the locker room door was for her.

I haven't had another massage yet, but when I do I'm going to be much more careful to be sure I get the experience that I want.

Serge's story.

> What I like about my massage sessions with Debra is that they are so well integrated. I always learn or experience a new relaxation technique when I go for a massage. Over the past couple of years as a client, I've experienced traditional deep muscle massage, craniosacral techniques, aromatherapy, ear coning, "knuckle" massage, rice sock-neck relief, and meditation. I feel so refreshed and renewed after each session I have with Debra. I also talk about various things with her that I wouldn't normally talk about with some of my closest friends. I feel I can confide in my massage therapist about some of my most troublesome concerns. Massage is one of the best ways I know to truly treat yourself and give your body the care and nurturing it deserves.

> I try to go at least on a monthly basis, and I find I look forward to it each month, more so than an upcoming party, a meeting with a close friend, or a Sunday hike. I recommend massage for everyone in order to achieve higher well-being and good health. I don't feel like I'd be a "complete" person without experiencing it regularly.

Ray's story.

> When I visit Debra on massage day, I feel like I am arriving at the airport, waiting to go on a relaxing vacation to an exotic destination. All I can think about is relaxing, unwinding, becoming one with myself.

> For me massage represents a regrouping—getting in touch with myself, not just physically but spiritually and

emotionally. Before Debra starts, my body feels tight, stressed, energy choked, and starved. Massage helps balance out and correct the energy I feel within me that is begging to be stirred and released. Massage for me is my tune-up for my internal and external energies. When I am tuned up, my body, mind, spirit, and life circumstances tend to work and flow better. Massage helps to help me perform as a person at my most optimum levels.

Before getting my first massage, I thought like a lot of people that massage was something that movie stars and people with a lot of money and time on their hands did to pass the time away and have fun. After receiving massage off and on for ten years now, I know why movie stars and the like get massages—massage helps to de-stress oneself and helps to make the person whole and complete again. My wife and I have a dream that if we had the money and time we would hire a full time massage therapist and start every day with a meditation and massage session.

Mark B's story (The Good Soldier).

The starting point was when I woke up with what felt like a knife in my rhomboids going through my right clavicle, and I thought this is gonna be a long day. It hurt so bad it made me sweat. I had to figure out how to get out of bed; had to bring my legs up and kick myself out of bed. Heat from the shower wouldn't take away the pain. Limped to work and had to figure out how to do dentistry without bending my head and back. I define crises as not being able to work, and I was getting there.

I called a friend to tell her what trouble I was in, and she called the chiropractor next door to fit me in their schedule. They couldn't, but referred me to a massage therapist that would see me that evening.

Debra had just moved from one place to a new office that afternoon. There were still boxes unpacked and the office was unpainted. I took enough aspirin to slough-off my stomach lining to make it until 5:00 p.m. I had a lot of apprehension about the whole thing—*ick*! I don't want to take my clothes off in front of someone...what if I end up with a tattoo? What did I know about massage—most of what I knew involved my '69 Firebird in high school. It was dark early since it was November, and that made it even spookier because I had to go in the dark.

Showed up, went through the door and met Debra; she actually wasn't Freddy Krueger with a chain saw. I explained my woes and troubles, and Debra told me what the rules were. I hurt like hell but didn't let my denial show. Then she left and I stripped down to my boxers, and Debra got to work.

So I spent the next hour getting evaluated—Debra spent an hour figuring out what my fat, lumpy body was doing. When we were all done, she told me to take it easy and get up slowly. Had to get up on my knees first before getting off the table. I was surprised I wasn't cured in one hour—apparently I needed more sessions.

Debra gave me exercises to do at home. At the end of this professional discussion, I told her I was a good soldier and Debra said, "That's why you're here." No tattoos!

Christi's story.

As a counselor for foreign exchange students, I must be constantly attuned to my needs for the gifts that rejuvenate, re-create, and reawaken my spirit. Quick fixes are easy, but not satisfying. I have come to a point in my life where I recognize junk food cravings and impulse buying for what they are: symptoms. Symptoms of spiritual starvation. Instead, I now seek things to quell the real hunger.

Everyone has a secret nurturing recipe. My ingredients vary. Sometimes my self-time includes a perfect forty-five minute steaming cup of chai on a rainy night, a favorite but vague poem rediscovered in a thick book, story hour on the radio, daydreaming on the couch for hours, a son born whole and vibrant.

The most recent addition to my self-care list is my monthly massage. Massage is a cure, salve, a potion that revives and nourishes me. Massage gives me permission to take without worry. Taking time. Taking mental space. Taking pleasure.

Without the balance, without the refueling, without the nourishment, I cannot continue to give. Massage clears the way to giving. It centers me in the now.

It stabilizes my feet so that I walk with purpose, with direction.

This is the symbiosis. This is the recipe. This is the balance.

Sheri's story.

A couple of weeks after my car accident—where my sternum, skin, and membrane were bruised and injured by my seat belt, and I had a pretty good case of whip-lash—I went to Reeni for a massage. (I actually used the Christmas present gift certificate from my husband for it!) She made me nice and warm, there was a soft wa-terfall nearby, and she gently massaged my head, neck, shoulders, and my upper chest. My WHOLE body melt-ed. Utter pleasure!

I received my next massage in the winter on a cold, gray frigid day. My massage therapist had a heater under the table, and mega soft blankets under me and on top of me. Yet another great massage.

Teresa's story.

Massage helps me to stay physically, mentally, and emo-tionally healthy. Like many people, I lead a busy life, full of activities, commitments, and responsibilities. I carry a lot of tension in my shoulders, which results in fre-quent headaches. Nothing relieves my stress like a good massage.

When I receive a massage, I experience three distinct phases:

Phase One: My mind and body slow down and begin to relax. There are few other times in my life when this happens.

Phase Two: My thoughts, body, and emotions all come together as I relax even deeper and begin to enjoy the release of tension.

Phase Three: Near the end of the massage, I feel physically relaxed, mentally at peace, and emotionally free. I feel wonderful about the fact that I have taken the time to look after and take care of myself.

Tom's story.

I am an artist in Connecticut. In recent months, I have had the opportunity to be involved in massage therapy, which has been a wonderful experience. I say therapy because that is what it has proven to be for me.

I previously had only two other massages in my life, which, as I remember, were nice at the time. I find that an ongoing relationship with massage does move me into a different place with it. Massage has not only allowed me to find a new physical freedom but also an inner soul-spirit kind of freedom.

It has shown that I can make a connection to my physical body, honor who I am, and know myself at different levels of consciousness.

Marilyn's story.

I've been very lucky to have known Debra Ty all her life, and recently she and her family visited me in Florida. Unfortunately, a week before they arrived, I had some minor surgery and was pretty uncomfortable. I called my doctor to let him know how uncomfortable I was, and he prescribed a new medication in hopes that it would make me feel better. The new medication turned out to be a disaster. My back began cramping, my hands were cramping, and my right leg ached. I didn't know what was happening to me, and I was scared.

Debra, her mother, and I were sitting in my living room chatting while I was trying to act as though I was fine. Debra, however, noticed me moving my leg back and forth and asked what was going on. I explained what was happening, and she came over, took my foot in her hands, and started working her magic. And magic is the only way for me to describe what happened over the next few minutes because the ache in my leg went away. I don't mean it got a little better—the ache was completely gone. MAGIC. I don't completely understand craniosacral therapy, but it works.

Later in the weekend, Debra had me lie on my back on my bed and she took my head in her hands (my back was still cramping), and I could actually feel what can only be described as a sort of electricity leaving my body through my tailbone. Yup, her hands were under my head on my neck, and the bad stuff left my body through my tailbone. Again, MAGIC. My back stopped cramping and I felt much, much better.

I had previously turned my nose up at any laying-on-of-the-hands kind of therapy, but I'm definitely a believer now. Again, I don't know how it works, but it works. To Debra, it's not magic because she's had years and years of training and knows exactly what to do, but to me it's still magic. Thank you, Debra.

Kathy's story.
Until a few years ago, I would get a massage once or twice a year, and I viewed each one as a treat or an indulgence. In my mid-forties I started experiencing lower-back and hip pain after playing tennis. It got so bad that I was worried that I would have to stop playing a game that I truly loved.

In desperation, I looked for solutions that would alleviate the pain. In addition to starting a regular yoga practice, I found a massage therapist that combined massage and craniosacral therapy to correct my alignment and work my tight muscles. What a relief! I have been getting regular monthly massages for five years now, still playing tennis with virtually no pain.

I now see regular massage as a necessity, something I must do for myself so that I can lead the type of active life I desire.

Patrice's story.

> My story began about fifteen years ago. As part of a routine checkup for obtaining my Youth Bus Driver's license, my physician's assistant found a cyst on my left ovary. She promptly referred me to an eminent oncologist in Irving, California—a three-hour drive from my home. Two weeks later, lying in the specialist's exam room, he did indeed verify the cyst and he casually informed me that I should "have both ovaries removed—and, certainly, it was best to have a complete hysterectomy!" At my age, about forty, I did not really need any of that equipment anyway. I dressed, got in my car and quickly drove home wishing I didn't have to pay his ridiculous fee for advising such a radical approach. Needless to say, I never consulted with this eminent oncologist ever again!

> Shocked and worried, I began to consider why my otherwise-very-strong body was treating me this way. Many hours of thought and meditation brought me to a place where I decided I wasn't paying enough attention to the wonders of my body, to how well it had served me, and the tenderness it deserved. I set about exploring the options for my situation. Foremost was my decision to "get in touch" with my body and appreciate my womanness and monthly menstrual cycles. I began conversations with dear friends, and it became apparent that my friends, too, had similar internal longings in regard to their bodies.

> We began casually meeting on weekends, and soon decided to form a women's group and build ourselves a

"moon lodge" for retreat and reflection. In the following months, we spent our time building a model of our project, forming our tight little group, and speaking our intentions. We built a beautiful lodge in the desert behind my house, and spent many long hours digging, stacking, mixing clay, and hanging the roof. We ventured to the high country for long willow branches meant for the roof structure. We dragged eucalyptus logs in for the walls, and we sought out local mud for chinking. We brought our special ornaments and our blood to the lodge. Many, many happy, sad, and painful hours were absorbed in the lodge, and in our singing, crying, dancing around the fire, and telling our own personal stories. Our bond of sisterhood became deep and lasting.

At the beginning of this process, Debjil (a nickname of Debra's) and I connected and began our "Purple Reiki"—the genius of the endeavor. The deep sensations and dreamworld that I experienced while in Debjil's studio, gave birth to a vision and affirmed my desire to connect with my body. Over many months, my mind and body were loosened and released to help me find whatever center existed for me. Through additional massage sessions, years of strangled emotions and fears would arise and eventually fall away.

I remember one massage session with another friend, Marla, an expert therapist, as she began stroking and kneading my sore body. After only a few minutes, I was completely overcome with tears streaming down my cheeks, an uncontrolled complete release of some mighty tensions in my body. It was heavenly. I knew that massage had to become a part of my wellness program.

I made my budget at the time to include an hourly massage every Monday night. Over the past twenty years, massage came and went in my life, and I strive to keep it as a constant part of my wellness routine. Sometimes I let it fall to the back burner and forget how critical it is for my mind and body. Then I get a massage and remember all the deep and delirious places it touches in my body and mind.

Another time in my life that was particularly sad and deeply emotional for me was a time a few years before our moon lodge group. Again, massage therapy helped me regain my life.

At the time, I was living with a man for about two years, and working myself into the ground and raising my two-year-old son. This man and I had been off and on again, and we just moved into our new home on two acres in the desert. We had decided to marry and were purchasing the home together. After a residence of only two months, he left for work the morning after Thanksgiving with his parents and family, never to come home again; he was struck on his motor cycle and later died from the injuries.

Devastated, alone, and miserable, I trudged on for several months. Friends encouraged me to try to move on. I decided to book a massage at the local health club with a person I did not know, but I had heard positive referrals. A little anxious, I showed up for the massage. An expert therapist began to unravel my torn body and mind in his gentle but strong hands. Again, pure heaven. Booked myself every week. This massage session continues, on and off through the years. After weeks of convincing this massage therapist that he wasn't breaking the professional decorum of our client and therapist relationship, we began to date. About a year later, we were married. That was twenty-five years ago.

Cecelia's story (As told by me, the author).

At the time of this story, my friends were raising two children, ages five and seven. My husband and I were close friends with their family, and we visited with them most Saturday evenings. The children—Carlos was seven, and Cecelia, five—were like most siblings; sometimes they fought and sometimes they got along spectacularly. This particular Saturday evening, they were not getting along well, and they began to hit each other even after being separated and punished for quarreling. There were continual tears, retaliations, and physical and emotional wounds.

Bedtime came around, and they did not want to go to bed, of course. I told Cecelia—who loves foot massage—that if she got into bed, I would give her a foot massage to help her fall asleep, and she agreed happily. While I massaged her feet, she told me about her day, and then she said, "When you are finished massaging my feet, I want you to massage Carlos's feet because he would really like this."

Cecelia amazed me. I watched her get the worst of her brother's verbal and physical abuse that evening, but after a little time out with my nurturing and kindness, she wanted the same for Carlos, who had been hurting her.

May massage do the same for you and for anyone you know; and may it do the same for everyone.

Chapter 15:
Your Massage Story

Each person has a story to tell. As well, we like to read stories, especially if the events are familiar to us or if they hit home in some way. So I leave space in the following pages for *your* story, thinking that, perhaps, someone else's narrative has inspired one within you. If you are gifting an individual you know with this book, surprise the receiver with your massage experience; and if space allows, leave room for the individual's own story. Maybe this book is yours to keep; if this is the case, enjoy writing your story for yourself. Furthermore, I encourage you to read and re-read the information in this book, and enjoy it at your leisure.

Your Massage Story

Massage Bloopers

The unexpected happens despite our best efforts, education, and experience. Here then are examples of humorous and embarrassing situations that took place on the massage table:

Blooper #1. It is always the unexpected witty comeback—the *repartee*—that helps to lighten absorbing moments. My first blooper happened during my first year as a massage therapist and at the very beginning of the client's massage, and it went like this:

> I started with a vigorous, stimulating, and thorough scalp massage. When I stopped, my client declared: "You know that's got to feel good if I let you undo my $50 cut and style."

Blooper #2. To help my process of getting over what I had done in the first blooper, I shared the story with a friend, Marla, who was also a massage therapist. In return, she disclosed one of her own bloopers, which I paraphrase here:

> As Marla was massaging her client's arms and hands, she took the time to savor and complete the stroke by ending all the way past the fingertips, only to be left with the client's artificial fingernail in her own hand.

Blooper #3. Though lengthy and not as lighthearted as the first two bloopers, this situation conveys how trust and friendship within the massage setting may develop over time and become an added benefit for both the therapist and client. This is what happened:

For about four years, Dennis had been coming to see me for his monthly massages. It gradually became part of our routine to allow time to chat before his session began, as we do not chat during the massage.

On one particular visit, the day's rambling was about the way people interpret what we say that is different than what we intend, no matter how clearly we believe to have communicated our thoughts. We both found this realization to be perplexing and, at times, frustrating, and we proceeded to share our experiences with this in mind, settling into our usual humorous dynamic.

After we finished chatting, Dennis made his way onto the massage table. About halfway through I asked him to turn onto his back, and I inquired how he was doing. "Good, so far," he replied. *So far*, how odd, I thought. Did Dennis not expect the rest of the massage to be good? After all, he had received years of beneficial massages from me. Anyway, I continued his massage by dropping essential oils on his chest, and as I was putting the bottle back on the counter, he cupped his eye with one hand and said, "Ouch, you got me in the eye!"

Never in my twenty-three years of therapy had this happened, so I felt terrible and concerned; essential oils are highly concentrated and could cause harm if used incorrectly. I handed Dennis his handkerchief so he could blot the affected eye, and I retrieved some eye drops from my desk drawer. His eyes were closed so tightly from the pain, I was not sure the drops were flushing his eye. I left the room and soaked a paper towel with water, and then dabbed the towel over his eye. Although he was still in pain, the wet towel helped just enough to open his eye slightly for another try with the drops, and Dennis asked to keep a fresh towel on his eye since it felt soothing to him.

The stinging subsided gradually, but the soreness remained while he was there. We continued with the massage, and after some time had passed, he asked me how he was going to explain the incident to his wife, because he was "coming home a pirate." This was just the comic relief I needed, but I retorted: "And not a good one at that, with a white rag instead of a black patch." The banter continued. "I suppose," I added, "when I heard you say the massage was 'good, so far,' I played right into doubts, which I assumed you had about the second half of the massage being good, too." To this, Dennis replied, "Is that how you interpreted what I said?" So there we were, right back with our initial conversation that preceded his massage.

The following day, I called Dennis at work to see how his eye was doing. "He is only half blind today," was his usual joking response; but he also said that it meant a great deal that I checked in on him. Well, how could I not? I care about his well-being. In the end, our unfortunate mishap with the oils strengthened our trust and friendship even more.

A Sacred Mission

We have been called to a most sweet work...a high calling...
a sacred mission.
Focus your mind inward now...to a soft place in your heart.
Come with me and sink into this vision...
We sit in a pool of beauty...we are filled up now...
And we see a stream of beings come to us to refresh themselves...
to lighten their heaviness...to remind them of their peace...
to unwind the twists and knots of pain and habit...
They come to be honored...to have someone spend an hour
on them...
just to receive...for many this is the only time they just receive.
They come to remember who they are...to feel themselves.
They thank us and we remind them it is their body that feels...
our hands give them a way to feel themselves.
They come for peace...for rest from a world of responsibility.
They come for someone to listen to them...to be known...to be
accepted.
They come to sleep, perhaps to dream. How precious. Have you
ever gone to a stranger's room and fallen asleep in their hands?
What trust! What trust they find in us.
They come to us for a safe place...a sanctuary...to let down
their guard of watchfulness...to soften...to open...to rest...
to refresh...to re-nourish on every level.
And we attend to them.
Truly we are the hands of healing...
the hands that bring peace...
the hands of tenderness...
the hands that are healing our world.
We nourish our bodies with good food, exercise and loving touch.

We nourish our minds with lovely visions and enriching thoughts.
We nourish our hearts with radiant good feelings.
We nourish our spirits with knowing our connection to Wholeness,
Oneness and Peace.
We nourish those who come to us.
Today we nourish ourselves and commit to filling ourselves full.

~Sandra Marak
Wholistic Health Facilitator
Hospice Coach
Peacemaker

Selected Bibliography

I have given you a basic start to understanding what massage has to offer and how it affects the body, mind, emotions, and spirit; yet there is so much more to learn. If you would like to expand and deepen your knowledge in these areas, you may find the following books helpful:

Barral, Jean-Pierre, D.O. *Understanding The Messages of Your Body: How to Interpret Physical and Emotional Signals to Achieve Optimal Health*. Berkeley, Ca.: North Atlantic, 2007.

Becker, Robert, and Gary Selden. *The Body Electric: Electromagnetism And The Foundation Of Life*. New York: William Morrow, 1985.

Benjamin, Ben, and Gale Borden, M.D. *Listen To Your Pain*. New York: Penguin Books, 1984.

Claire, Thomas. *Body Work: What Type of Massage to Get And How to Make the Most of It*. Laguna Beach, Ca.: Basic Health Publications, 2006.

Downing, George. *The Massage Book: 25ᵗʰ Anniversary Edition*. New York: Random House, 1972.

Dychtwald, Ken. *Body-Mind*. New York: Pantheon Books, 1986.

Essential Science Publishing, compiler. *Essential Oils Desk Reference, 4th ed.* [Orem, UT?]: Essential Science Publishing, 2009.

Kaptchuk, Ted J., O.M.D. *The Web That Has No Weaver: Understanding Chinese Medicine.* New York: McGraw-Hill, 2000.

Maxwell-Hudson, Clare. *The Complete Book of Massage.* New York: Random House, 1988.

Montagu, Ashley. *Touching: The Human Significance of the Skin.* New York: Harper & Row, 1986.

Moore, Thomas. *Care of the Soul In Medicine: Healing Guidance for Patients, Families, and the People Who Care for Them.* Carlsbad, Ca.: Hay House, 2010.

Mumford, Susan. *The New Complete Guide to Massage.* New York: Plume/Penguin Group, 2007.

Myss, Caroline, Ph.D. *Anatomy of the Spirit: The Seven Stages of Power and Healing.* New York: Three Rivers Press, 1996.

National Center for Complementary and Alternative Medicine. "What Is Complementary and Alternative Medicine?" NCCAM. http://nccam.nih.gov/health/whatiscam/

National Certification Board for Therapeutic Massage & Bodywork. "Code of Ethics," revised October 2008 (Part XII). NCBTMB. http://www.ncbtmb.org/about _code_of_ethics.php (accessed October 6, 2011)

Stein, Diane. *Essential Reiki: A Complete Guide to an Ancient Healing Art.* New York: Crossing Press, 1995.

Thie, John F., and Matthew Thie. *Touch For Health: The Complete Edition.* Camarillo, Ca.: DeVorss & Company, 2005.

Upledger, John E., D.O., O.M.M. *Your Inner Physician and You: Craniosacral Therapy and Somatoemotional Release.* Berkeley, Ca.: North Atlantic Books, 1997.

Worwood, Susan E., and Valerie Ann Worwood. *Essential Aromatherapy: A Pocket Guide to Essential Oils and Aromatherapy.* Novato, Ca.: New World Library, 2003.

Other Resources

The National Center for Complementary and Alternative Medicine (NCCAM):
(888) 644-6226 or online at http://nccam.nih.gov/

CAM (Complementary and Alternative Medicine) is a branch of The National Institute for Health in Maryland: (301) 496-4000 or online at http://www.nih.gov

American Massage Therapy Association (AMTA): 1-877-905-0577 or online at http://www.amtamassage.org

About the Author

In 1987, Debra Ty completed her Holistic Health Practitioner's training from the International Professional School of Bodywork (IPSB) in San Diego, California. Concurrently, she obtained a Bachelor of Arts degree from the University for Humanistic Studies in Del Mar, also in California, studying the psyche and its relationship to the body. She holds a certification with the National Certification Board for Therapeutic Massage & Bodywork (NCBTMB), and is a member of the American Massage Therapy Association (AMTA) and Associated Psychotherapists of Vermont (APOV).

Debra has a private practice in Vermont, and teaches the MELT Method, and other self-care topics.

Debra lives with her partner Ron and her cat Sir Oreo in Vermont, her birth state.

Visit her website at: http://www.acenterforcaring.com